SURVIVING LEUKEMIA

Surviving Leukemia

A PRACTICAL GUIDE

Dr. Robert Patenaude

KEY PORTER BOOKS

Canadian Cataloguing in Publication Data

Patenaude, Robert, 1957-
    Surviving leukemia : a practical guide

Translation of: Survivre à la leucémie

ISBN 1-55263-046-3

1. Leukemia–Treatment. 2. Blood–Diseases–Treatment. 3. Bone marrow
–Transplantation. 4. Oncology–Dictionaries–Health. 5. Patenaude, Robert,
1957 -   . 6. Leukemia–Patients–Quebec (Province)–Biography. I. Title.

RC643.P3713 1999   616.99'41906   C98-932999-2

Canadä

We acknowledge the financial support of the Government of Canada through the Book Publishing Industry Development Program (BPIDP) for our publishing activities.

Key Porter Books Limited
70 The Esplanade
Toronto, Ontario
Canada M5E 1R2

www.keyporter.com

Electronic formatting: Susan Thomas
Design: Patricia Cavazzini

Printed and bound in Canada

99 00 01 02   6 5 4 3 2 1

Contents

Chapter 5   The Treatment of Blood Diseases 160

Chapter 6   Practical Advice for Patients 208

Acknowledgments

For special help and collaboration: Dr. E. Donnall Thomas, professor of medicine at the University of Washington.

For their scientific collaboration: Dr. Claude Perreault, hematologist, professor at the University of Montreal, and director of the Guy Bernier Research Center; Dr. Robert Bélanger, hematologist, professor at the University of Montreal, and director of the hematology department at Maisonneuve Rosemont Hospital; Dr. Giovani D'Angelo, coordinator of the hematologic laboratory of Maisonneuve Rosemont Hospital; Dr. Yvette Bony, pediatric hematologist, and professor at the University of Montreal; Dr. Denis Claude Roy, hematologist, professor at the University of Montreal, and director of the autologous bone marrow program at Maisonneuve Rosemont Hospital; and Dr. Lambert Busque, hematologist, professor at the University of Montreal, and director of the molecular hematology department at Maisonneuve Rosemont Hospital.

For special support and trust in this project: Jocelyne Morrissette, M. Jacques Fortin and all the group of Quebec/Amerique Editions; and Mary Ann McCutcheon, Clare McKeon and all the group at Key Porter Books.

Very special thanks to my friends and colleagues at work for their patience and understanding and to my family, who trusted, helped and supported me for all these years in such wonderful projects: writing books.

Special thanks to my mother Jeannine, my sister Line and my two little nieces Amelie and Emmanuelle, to Dominique Croteau and his family for their constant support and help, to Serge Dubuc and his family, who are old-time friends, and to Michelle Coudé-Lord, for such good advice.

Preface

Dr. E. Donnall Thomas is professor emeritus at the University of Washington. He has devoted his life to leukemia research, particularly in the area of bone marrow transplants. In 1990, Dr. Thomas received the Nobel Prize for medicine for his collective work on bone marrow transplants.

I personally owe my own recovery to the work of Dr. Thomas. In 1981, he was the first to perform early bone marrow grafts on patients with chronic myeloid leukemia. Having read my first book Dr. Thomas agreed to write the preface for Surviving Leukemia, for which I am deeply grateful.

In the 1950s, the first bone marrow grafts were attempted on humans. Following heavy doses of chemotherapy and radiotherapy, bone marrow from a healthy donor was transferred to a patient, but the success rate was low. The best results were obtained when grafts were performed between identical twins (syngeneic transplants).

Allogeneic marrow grafts (involving donors who are not genetically identical) were limited by very serious complications such as the graft being rejected, the graft reacting to the host and the development of severe infections.

In the 1960s, studies were conducted on animals (mice, rats and dogs) in order to better understand the importance of organ typing between donors and recipients. By the end of the 1960s, we were able to define the different types of white blood cells in humans: this research gave birth to HLA (Human Leucocyte Antigen) groups. From that moment on, we could identify individuals within the same family who would be compatible for bone marrow transplants.

In the years that followed, we demonstrated that it was possible to cure patients with myelosuppression and advanced leukemia.

Over the last ten years, the number and types of diseases that can be treated through bone marrow transplants have increased dramatically and recovery rates have exceeded all predictions.

We owe this success to the work of many researchers and well-trained medical teams. Recently, the appearance of non-related bone marrow donor banks has allowed several patients without a family member donor to receive a bone marrow transplant.

Some patients without a donor can even be treated by transplanting their own bone marrow (autologous graft). A bone marrow graft is a complicated treatment involving several medical therapies such as chemotherapy, radiotherapy, immunology and the treatment of infectious diseases. Transplant centers have specialized nursing and medical staff, highly skilled in recognizing complications arising from a transplant and in quickly beginning treatment.

In today's high-tech medical world, it is not surprising patients and their families have difficulty in understanding everything that is happening around them. Most books on the types and treatment of blood diseases are very technical because they are written for nurses and doctors working in this field. It is, therefore, with great pleasure that we welcome *Surviving Leukemia* by Dr. Patenaude.

This highly comprehensible work will help all patients and their families.

Dr. E. Donnall Thomas

Dr. Claude Perreault, a hematologist, is a pioneer in the field of bone marrow grafting in Canada. Today, as head of the Guy Bernier Research Center in Montreal, he devotes his time to bone marrow transplant research. Dr. Perreault has made numerous discoveries in the field of immunology as it relates to transplants, for which he is recognized internationally by his peers.

For many readers, Robert Patenaude's book will initially be a mine of information on blood and blood diseases, especially since this unique book is accessible to non-medical readers. Fortunately, it is this and more as the teachings of the doctor mesh with the reflections of the man.

For most of its history, medicine was an art. After having lost its "secrets" and having amassed a considerable amount of knowledge, medicine has become a science whose rapid and exciting progress cannot be discussed without also defining its limits. Robert Patenaude succeeds, without any smugness or triumphalism, in painting a picture that accurately reflects the latest in hematology, without forgetting that, for some readers, the relationship with blood disease is not just theoretical. For them in particular, as well as for all others, reading the thoughts of this man will be a source of inspiration.

Dr. Claude Perreault

Introduction

It is 1979. In a corridor in Emergency, crowded with patients, a doctor is speaking to a young woman sitting on a stretcher:

"The disease you have, leukemia, is terminal. This means that it can't be cured."

The young woman's face drops. Her sadness and outrage are palpable.

In 1982, in the corridor in Emergency, overflowing with patients, a doctor is talking with a young man sitting on a stretcher:

"The only treatment that has any hope of curing you is a bone marrow transplant."

"What are the odds?" asks the patient.

"Thirty percent. It's not a lot, but it's better than nothing."

The young man is sad and outraged, but his eyes are full of hope. He announces: "O.K., let's do it." I was this patient.

In 1999, in the same corridor in Emergency, still packed with patients, a doctor is speaking with a young woman sitting on a stretcher:

"You have a type of leukemia, however, thanks to bone marrow grafting, we can now cure more than 70% of all patients."

As you can see, the treatment of the different types of leukemia has considerably and quickly evolved since 1979. So much so that today, many types are now curable.

In 1998, more than 10,000 new cases of malignant blood disease were recorded in Canada: leukemia, lymphoma, myeloma, aplasia and many others. These diseases attack both children and adults.

For many patients, leukemia is incomprehensible, as it does not always display symptoms that can be touched or seen, such as lumps or lesions. It often spreads to organs that we know little of or which are rarely discussed, such as the spleen, lymph nodes and bone marrow.

This work explains, in simple terms, these different diseases and tries to describe the psychological stages that the patient goes through from the moment the disease is diagnosed until it is cured.

A concluding chapter offers practical advice for patients currently undergoing treatment. Refer as well to the series of photographs illustrating the principal malignant blood diseases. In conclusion, a glossary provides definitions of the main medical terms used in oncology.

I wish you an enjoyable read.

"Doctor, You Have Leukemia"   I

Hope is the magical link
that takes us by the hand
and leads us to healing.

Having gone through a bone marrow transplant in 1982, when I was a second-year medical student, I am eager to tell you my story, enriched with the experiences of other people who have also undergone transplants and whom I know well because of my profession and my commitment to the fight against cancer.

I have included quotes and poems throughout my book to make it easier to understand what patients and their families experience throughout an illness and its treatment.

The Crushing Blow

October 1981

In one of the university's laboratories, second-year medical students set up their microscopes. In the meantime, the white-haired professor explained the experiment in store:

"First, you must extract a drop of blood by pricking the tip of your finger. Then you dilute the drop with a solution of water and salts and delicately place it on the microscope's slide. Be quick, because outside the body white blood cells survive for only a few minutes.

"Then you add bacteria and, after adjusting your microscope to magnify four hundred times, move the slide under the objective and try to find the white blood cells. You will observe phagocytosis, which as you know is the ability of white blood cells to recognize bacteria and eat them.

"For this particular experiment, you will be working in groups of three."

As usual, I worked with two friends, Serge and Stephan. We drew straws to see who would be the guinea pig and I was the lucky winner. We followed the method described by our professor and looked at our test.

"I must be lucky; I see six white blood cells," I said.

Stephan took a look and added, "Your white blood cells are lazy, pal, they're not eating any bacteria."

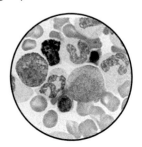

After a bit of joking, Serge took a look through the microscope. "Hey, Bob, he's right. Your white blood cells are lazy. And when I move the slide around, I can see even more of them. That's strange."

Since I had the flu, we concluded that the number of white blood cells had increased because of the temporary infection in my body. Serge pricked his own finger for a drop of blood and we began the experiment again. Serge's blood cells were fewer in number and efficient in eating bacteria.

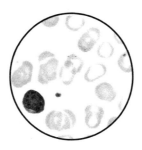

November 1981

The weather had turned cold and all the leaves had fallen from the trees weeks earlier. I was seated with 209 other students in a poorly ventilated and overheated room. Impatiently, we awaited the end of the 11:30 class: every day, we got together to play one sport or another. Hockey season had started and we were scheduled to play our first game against the third-year team. I love every sport, but my favorite is hockey. When the class ended—at last—I was quick to leave. A secretary approached me in the halls:

"Are you Robert Patenaude?"

"Yes."

"The doctor at the university clinic has been trying to reach you for two weeks—you aren't home very often! He wants to see you as soon as possible."

"Why?"

"I don't know, but it seems to be important."

"Okay, I'll go to see him next week."

"No, he wants to see you this afternoon."

"Okay, then, I'll go to see him after the hockey game."

One month earlier, each medical student had been given a complete physical examination, including blood tests and a lung X-ray. We had to submit to these tests before we could do our internships in hospitals.

When the hockey game was over, I went to the clinic, convinced that I had a sexually transmitted disease (STD); still, I had no symptoms. The doctor asked me a number of questions:

"Do your bones hurt?"

"No."

"Do you bleed often, do you bruise easily?"

"No."

"Have you lost weight?"

"No."

"Do you sweat at night?"

Joking, I answered, "That depends on whether or not I'm sleeping alone."

He examined me and added, "The examination is normal, except that your spleen is enlarged. Don't engage in any violent sports like hockey or football until further notice; your spleen could rupture and that may lead to abdominal bleeding."

"So, what's wrong with me, Doctor? Is it an STD?"

"No, it's a blood problem. But before I can tell you more, I'd like you to go to a hematology department at a teaching hospital. I made an appointment for you for tomorrow morning."

The next day I went to the hospital's emergency ward; a very nice but obviously overworked nurse assigned me to stretcher thirty-seven and told me: "You'll have to put on a hospital gown; if you need anything, just call me."

Intrigued, I asked, "How many sick people are waiting in the corridors?"

"For now, things are quiet; there are about sixty. But on the weekend there'll be about ninety."

I was flabbergasted. I put on the horrendous hospital gown and sat down, looking at the comings and goings. The place looked like a subway station from hell. Decidedly, my baptism of fire in the medical system wasn't like anything I could have imagined. At last, a hematology student came to examine me.

"I'll be doing blood tests, a bone marrow puncture, and a bone biopsy."

"Why? Is all this really necessary?"

"Yes, if we want to be sure of your diagnosis, the tests are crucial."

"What exactly is wrong with me?"

"We'll do the tests and we'll talk about it this afternoon."

After a bit of pain in the lower back area and a great deal of sweat, I was finished with the tests, and the samples were sent to the laboratory.

Around four o'clock in the afternoon, two students and a hematologist returned. The first student outlined my medical history and all three discussed the results of the blood test and bone marrow puncture. After a few seemingly endless minutes, at last they arrived at a diagnosis. The hematologist told me: "Doctor, you have chronic myelogenous leukemia. Basically, the disease is cancer of the white blood cells; they multiply and prevent the growth of healthy blood cells."

I was speechless, my throat went dry, tears came to my eyes. But I wanted to hide my emotions. Then the hematologist gave me more details on the disease.

"The average survival time is two to three years, but the disease develops well; in other words, it doesn't cause any physical problems. To stabilize it, we administer oral chemotherapy: the medication doesn't cause any hair loss and doesn't have any side effects."

After a few moments of thought he added, "I would prefer to keep you under observation until tomorrow morning, then you can go home. Do you have any questions?"

In a choking voice I asked, "So, I really do have leukemia?"

"Yes, you really have leukemia."

Suddenly, I remembered the phagocytosis laboratory experiment we had done one month earlier. Although we hadn't drawn any conclusions, we had noticed the high number of white cells in my blood and their inability to eat bacteria—a warning sign of leukemia. But at the time, we lacked the knowledge to make a diagnosis.

With an increasingly heavy heart, pounding harder and harder in my chest, I continued, not without some difficulty: "Well! Can I have a room for the night?"

"Impossible. You have to spend at least three or four days in 'purgatory' before you can hope to go to heaven. Every room is taken; I'd

19

like to give you one, but I can't. The 'hotel' is full; you'll have to spend the night here."

I asked again, "Are you sure I have leukemia?" The doctor nodded in the affirmative, but did not say a word.

And then all three moved away from me, discussing their next case.

I felt bad and guilty about this last question and the reaction of the doctor. I told myself: Maybe I asked too many questions? Or maybe my doctor had too much work and was tired? I looked around; an old lady, who was sitting on a stretcher next to me receiving a blood transfusion, told me, "Don't worry, sometimes they make mistakes." I looked at her and said, "I hope so."

Shock and Denial

Shaken, I refused to believe the macabre news. Only twenty-four to thirty-six months to live? Come on, it makes no sense. It can't be happening to me. I'm sure that they're wrong. Anybody can make a mistake. I'll do other tests, I'll see another doctor....

Around midnight, I could no longer cope with the chaos of the emergency ward's hallways. My eyes were tired from the neon lighting and I was constantly bothered by other stretchers being pushed alongside mine, by the groans and complaints of other patients, by intercom messages. Sleep was unattainable even though I'd been given two sleeping pills. And because I'd been sweating all day, I wanted to take a shower; they told me I couldn't because it was too late. I decided to go home.

I called the nurse and told her: "I'm fed up, enough is enough. Tell the doctor that I'll call him tomorrow. I'm going home."

"You can't leave the hospital without the doctor's authorization; you have leukemia, it's serious, you have to stay here."

"I can't rest here; find me somewhere else to sleep or I'm leaving."

She returned to the nursing station to ask for her supervisor's help.

In a major hospital, supervising nurses usually have a great deal of experience; they have been working in "purgatory" for a number of years and they are not easily intimidated—not by patients, not by visitors, not by medical students. A few seconds later, she came to me, hands on her hips.

"What's wrong, young doctor?"

"I don't feel like staying here all night. I'm going home to sleep. And I don't care if you're not happy about that."

I must have been persuasive because she replied, "If you want to go, my friend, you'll have to sign a treatment refusal form; we don't want to be responsible for what happens to you."

Five minutes later I had signed all the papers and was ready to leave the hospital. A very elderly woman with a stomachache already had taken my place on stretcher thirty-seven. The nurses didn't even give me back the plastic hospital card with my name, address, and file number on it.

Outside, the sight of the winter's first snow, falling softly in oversized flakes, brought me some peace. I called a taxi. The Haitian driver, about fifty years old, looked at me in the rearview mirror and said, "You don't seem to be doing very well."

I told him my story, encouraged by his interest. At times, I can still see his wrinkled eyes looking back at me with sympathy.

When I finished telling him what had happened, he sighed a few times and then began to tell me about his childhood: "At twelve years old, I almost died of tuberculosis. In Haiti, at the time, many children died of the disease; they still do today, but in fewer numbers," he recounted somewhat reluctantly. "The village nurse had informed the family of my imminent death. My mother cried and prayed a lot. A few weeks went by and, little by little, I grew stronger. My old mother said it was a miracle."

"But leukemia is incurable."

"Trust in God and in life; you have to make room for miracles in your life. Sometimes the wind changes direction very, very quickly." Smiling, he added, "God didn't want me; he sent me back to earth to

21

resume my journey. Now I'm a taxi driver, in Montreal, in a snow-storm. Fate is unbelievable!"

He left me at my doorstep, handing me a slip of paper with his name and phone number on it. "If you want, we can go for coffee sometime; I'll introduce you to my wife and my five children."

He categorically refused payment for the ride and his car went on its way, slipping and sliding on the snow-covered road.

In the years to come, I visited Albert and his family time and time again in his Côte-des-Neiges neighborhood. He taught me that pride is never a good response in a difficult situation; it is much better to accept our limitations and the help of our friends, even if doing so isn't always easy.

Bargaining

The next day, I met with my doctor and told him candidly, "I agree to follow my treatment here, as long as I will not be hospitalized."

"All right, no problem," he answered.

So, like most people in the same circumstances, I was in the perfectly understandable bargaining stage. Often, patients try to ensure that they will get the best care, will experience less pain, and will live longer by using their good behavior as a bargaining tool with God, their loved ones, and the medical team. They promise to follow their treatment program scrupulously, to show more understanding toward others, to practice their religion faithfully. But they rarely fulfill their promises, and, of course, this only increases their guilt and their anxiety. Would I be any different?

Anger

> *When our loved ones complain of their misfortune or their illness, we extend our sympathy.*
> *When they assert themselves or show their strength and their independence by expressing their anger, we reject them.*

Dr. G.R. Bach, *Creative Aggression*

There are no words to describe the revolt, the helplessness, and the aggression that one feels when stricken by an incurable disease.

The subsequent months were very difficult, because at the outset of my treatment, no one ever referred to the possibility of a cure. I watched the weeks go by, like a countdown. I continued my studies, and medicine remained my main interest. However, I willingly skipped boring classes to get out into the fresh air, play a sport, or go for a beer at the campus café with my friends. My academic marks suffered, but I continued my studies all the same. It was all that mattered to me.

Why me? I used to say. I never did anything wrong, I always worked hard to get where I was. Why not a guy from a well-off family, living in a rich neighborhood, someone who has everything, someone who has never worked for anything?

I expressed my aggression through sports; I had begun to play hockey again since, with the medication, my spleen had returned to its normal size. Players from other faculties were on the receiving end of my anger and frustration. But my intolerance and impatience were also directed against friends and relatives, often in ordinary, everyday circumstances.

For example, since I was living with two other students in a medium-sized apartment, space was rather limited and we had to compromise. But I would be gruff or belligerent when dirty dishes piled up or when there was no more milk for breakfast or when I had no privacy. Luckily, my friends were very understanding and they didn't hold my occasional outbursts against me.

This isn't always the case. At times, when expressing anger or envi-ousness toward those who do not share their fate, patients are rejected by those close to them. Yet it is precisely at these times that they feel the keenest need to be listened to and understood. Their anger is jus-tified; after all, they are facing death. Anger is inevitable and it must be expressed.

Depression

Awareness that the illness is very real ("Yes, this is actually happening to me") often is accompanied by deep depression. Patients begin to regret their past, to mourn what they have not had the time to expe-rience, to withdraw from others. They may require the services of a psychiatrist or may need prescribed antidepressants.

Acceptance

Once past the stage of depression, patients usually succeed in accepting their illness; in other words, they relinquish their health. They accept seeing their bodies deteriorate, they accept living life day by day, never-theless staying hopeful. One saying teaches us that as long as there is life, there is hope. Personally, I tend to believe that as long as there is hope, there is life.

Long before my illness manifested itself, I took part in a competi-tion for students who wanted to do volunteer work in Africa during their summer holidays. The project was important to me and, in April 1982, I received a letter telling me that I had been accepted: "You will be flying to Yaounde, the capital of the Cameroon, next June 4th. From there, local representatives will direct you to a small dispensary for children, located two hundred kilometers to the south, in a village named Ebolowa."

The following week I received a telephone call from my doctor's secretary: the doctor wanted to meet with me as soon as possible. I figured that he had gotten wind of my project.

The next day, in his office, my doctor told me that an American study conducted by a Dr. Thomas of Seattle showed that bone marrow transplants could be practiced on patients suffering from chronic myelogenous leukemia. Although preliminary, results confirmed a 30 percent survival rate. Compatibility tests were conducted with my two sisters. Diane proved to be perfectly compatible.

From then on, I was convinced that I would be all right; my feeling wasn't rational, but rather a gut feeling, a sort of instinct for life that was never to leave me, a belief in miracles. And I kept repeating to myself the following words from Winston Churchill, spoken during the Second World War: "I will never surrender."

The Instinct to Live

The will to live is not a theoretical abstraction but a physiological reality with therapeutic characteristics.
Not all illnesses can be overcome, but more than a reasonable amount of people let illness ruin their lives. They yield to it needlessly because they neglect and weaken their power to stand up to it.
There is always a margin within which we can continue to live a life that is not deprived of sense, or even of joy, in spite of illness.

Norman Cousins, The Will to Heal

As soon as my doctor received the results of the compatibility tests, he wanted to perform the transplant before the summer.

"It's out of the question," I told him. "I'm leaving to work in Africa for three months, in a jungle dispensary. I wanted to tell you about it. I'm leaving on June 4."

He stared at me, astonished and overwhelmed by the news. "Are you joking? You can't be serious. Those countries are hard even on people who are in good health; for someone with leukemia, they would be a catastrophe. And the longer we put off your transplant, the lower the chance of success—statistics prove it."

The project meant too much to me to abandon it. If fate had put illness, Africa, and, soon, a transplant on my road, it had to bring me health as well.

After a lengthy discussion, we agreed to delay the transplant for a few months. In Africa, my chemotherapy treatments would be decreased and I would take a count of my white blood cells each week. If they went beyond a certain level, I would come home.

Africa

June 1982

The three-month interval in Africa was an absolutely invaluable human and social experience for me; on that continent—almost another planet—I met people who, despite abject poverty and even misery, were likable and capable of embracing life.

At six o'clock in the morning, I began my day by making my rounds to visit the hospitalized children, along with a Cameroonian nurse. Fifty or sixty small patients lay on rusted metal beds, aligned in three large, poorly ventilated, and stiflingly hot dormitories.

Mothers and other family members often slept on mats slid under the beds, since in these jungle hospitals families are responsible for feeding and washing the children. Parents often walk more than twenty kilometers to care for their little ones, and throughout their hospitalization, they stay with them.

In Africa, the main illnesses affecting children are infections. Cases of tuberculosis, meningitis, and dysentery were side by side with victims of road accidents and children suffering from serious malnutrition. Germs spread commonly, despite my efforts to isolate the most critical cases.

To care for these tiny patients, all we had were two or three microscopes and an outdated X-ray machine to help us make a diagnosis and determine a treatment. In most instances, the antibiotics administered to patients had expired several months previously. Yet, in my three months there I never heard one person complain, and the hospital enjoyed an excellent reputation since, according to the nurses, the situation was worse in other dispensaries.

After making my rounds, I assisted Dr. Sandiland, a seventy-two-year-old American surgeon who had come to Ebolowa forty years earlier. Unquestionably, Dr. Sandiland was a master surgeon, and his reputation extended as far as the Congo. A man of stature, he always had the serious air of a general who speaks only to give orders. In record time he operated on people suffering from intestinal cancers, perforated stomach ulcers, and multiple injuries incurred in road accidents (since Cameroonians drive dangerously on roads that are themselves dangerous). Despite outdated equipment, postoperative complications were rare.

My work with these children, the nurses, and Dr. Sandiland made me realize that even if my fate was sad, I had lived twenty-three beautiful years and had been very fortunate to be born in a country where we can do just about anything we want to, with minimal effort, compared to here. This experience opened my eyes to the dramatic situations of the world's most oppressed peoples, in countries where dictators, multinationals, and corrupt governments control wheat, medication, water, money, and much more. When I left the African continent, I promised myself that someday I would return.

I returned to Montreal ten kilograms lighter, having suffered three bouts of enteritis and one bout of malaria in Ebolowa. As soon as I arrived, I went to the hospital for a complete checkup and to gain a little weight before the bone marrow transplant, scheduled for October.

Money

At that time, a bone marrow transplant involved two or three months of hospitalization and three to six months of convalescence. Throughout this time, I would be forced to interrupt my studies.

A few days before my treatments began, I received a letter from the loans and bursaries division of the Department of Education. It read as follows:

> Mr. Patenaude:
>
> Since you have decided to interrupt your studies, we ask that you reimburse the bursary granted to you last September. The sum totals $803.55, plus $9.54 in interest, for a grand total of $813.09.
>
> In addition, we ask that you contact one of our auditors so that we can determine the terms for reimbursement of your loans, totalling $3,780.00.
>
> As you know, regulations stipulate that you must begin reimbursing loans six months after your studies have ended.

I read the letter at least three times. I was having a hard time believing my eyes. Now, on top of health problems, I had money problems! In 1982, you could live "comfortably" with a sum of $3,000 to $3,500 per year. With that amount we ate frugally (Kraft Dinner, vegetable stew, fish sticks with tomato sauce and onions, etc.), but we could go on a weekly outing (restaurants, the movies, a few beers at the end of a day) and we could live in an apartment (three of us in a medium-sized apartment in the basement of a building, dark and crisscrossed with heating system pipes). If I had no money, what would I do?

Since I didn't have rich parents or friends, I had to go begging to a civil servant at the Department of Education.

A Few Days Later

After a two-hour wait, among worried-looking students, most of whom were immigrants, all standing shoulder to shoulder, at last I was asked to step into the office of Mr. Roger V.

But Mr. Roger V. was on his "health break" for twenty minutes. Exactly twenty minutes went by, and Mr. Roger V. returned. He was in his early forties, with a bit of a paunch, and florid behind his big, thick glasses.

He sat down without a word, setting down a coffee cup emblazoned with "Old Orchard Beach, MAINE."

For a few seconds I traveled into the past, to a time several years ago when my family went on a seaside holiday. I loved the waves, loved how they went back and forth, digging trenches between my feet and swallowing up my dams and sand castles. It's funny how you can go so far away in so short a time!

"What's your permanent code?" mumbled Mr. Roger V. in a monotone voice, moving his cup to a mini hotplate and turning down his transistor radio.

"PATR 13075703," I said, giving him the code that identifies me in government files.

Mr. V. entered my number in the computer and, eyes riveted on the screen, asked, "What's wrong?"

I told him my whole story and closed by asking if I could reimburse my debt at a later date.

He looked at me, impassible. "Your parents can't help you?"

"Since my father had a heart attack, they've been on welfare."

"It's too bad, what's happening to you, but the rules are the same for everyone. You're leaving the university for more than one semester, so you're no longer considered to be a full-time student. You have to reimburse your loan; those are the rules."

"Yes, but ..."

"Listen, I don't make the rules. If you aren't happy, write to the department," interrupted the corpulent Mr. V., indicating that the meeting was over.

I left, noticing a sign at the door: Student Assistance Department!

Help from the Bank

No, a bank robbery wasn't what helped me. What did help was a tie, a well-ironed shirt, my friend Serge's suit coat, a "private school" haircut, and a small bending of the truth.

"Yes, Mr. Patenaude, I think we can lend you $5,000," said the bank manager as he handed me a very elaborate form I had to fill in. I did it on the spot.

Question 12: Have you received treatment for a cancer or a serious illness in the past five years?

I hesitated, weighing a lie and one year's peace against honesty and the resulting problems.

[ ] YES   [x] NO

We shook hands and he assured me that I would get a very quick answer. The next week, my loan was approved.

No, it wasn't honest, I admit, but I had no choice. But I have remained a loyal customer of the same bank and I do good business with it, and it does equally good business with me!

The Anxiety of Illness and Treatment

There can be several days, several weeks even, between the time you are told that you have some form of cancer and the time that treatment begins. It isn't rare for a bone marrow transplant candidate to wait two or three months before being hospitalized. This period is needed to prepare the transplant recipient and the donor; in cases of chronic myelogenous leukemia, the wait can extend to one year. During this period, many patients experience extreme stress; in this early stage it is good for patients to acquire the means to relax and to verbalize their fears and anxieties. Thus, they are better prepared for hospitalization.

This period is very difficult to live through because there is no miracle solution for confronting illness and death. We are afraid to speak out, afraid to face the situation head-on, afraid to bother others. We are constantly afraid. We think about our illness every minute of the day, and when we close our eyes at night, we would dearly love to believe that we will wake up and realize it's all a bad dream.

I was in a permanent state of apprehension, but I was not alone. For the past two months, my girlfriend Dominique had been sleeping beside me, accompanying me on this crazy earthly adventure.

As I cried over my lot in life, she was there to support me, despite my foul moods, my regression into childhood, my negotiations, my sadness, my anxieties, and my frustrations. Things certainly couldn't have been easy for her during that time.

Illness isn't any fun for anyone, not for spouses, families, and loved ones, nor for the patient. To weather the storm takes understanding, patience, and a deep closeness. After all, we are but human beings, with our weaknesses, our emotions, and our sensitivity.

The Transplant Period

A bone marrow transplant is a "second birth" that begins on the day you are hospitalized and ends when you return home.

First, doctors inserted a venous catheter at the thorax level. The plastic tube was used to give me the supplements that had to be administered directly into my blood, such as medication, transfusions, sugar- and protein-based liquids, and, in time, even bone marrow. The tube was my "umbilical cord" for the next eight weeks.

During the first week, I received radiotherapy and chemotherapy; since I am an anxious person, I experienced a great deal of nausea and vomiting, which is not the case with other people. In general, calm and relaxed patients react much better. Luckily for me, there are good antinausea medications that have no effect whatsoever on the success of the transplant.

The day before the operation, leafing through Ernest Hemingway's *The Old Man and the Sea*, I read: "Man never triumphs totally." And I told myself that the next day, as far as I was concerned, I would triumph over death thanks to a transplant of bone marrow from Diane; the next day, together we would push back by some ten years a meeting with death I see as inevitable.

Day 0

The day of the transplant is always a day charged with emotion. Some patients prefer to stay alone in their rooms; others spend the day on the phone, talking to relatives and friends, or greeting visitors. This is an exceptional time, and each person is free to live it as he or she sees fit.

6:15 a.m.
The sun has barely risen. Diane came to see me before going to the operating room. She didn't seem nervous.

"Don't worry, bro, your big sister will give you good cells and a couple of other good things besides. Maybe you'll be more like a woman and maybe you'll talk more after your transplant."

We laughed together for a few minutes, then she left me to go to the operating room.

9:15 a.m.

It was time for Diane to be anesthetized.

The operation consists of aspirating the bone marrow located in the donor's pelvis. The marrow looks like blood and is taken in several punctures using stiff needles and syringes. The process takes about two hours and is done under general anesthetic.

Today there's a new method—apheresis—in which the donor isn't needed in the operating room.

11:15 a.m.

The plastic bag containing one liter of Diane's bone marrow arrived. I touched it; it was still warm. It was filled with cells that would regenerate my blood and save my life.

Until that day, my blood was type O; now and for the rest of my days, my blood is type B, Diane's blood type.

12:15 p.m.

I received the bone marrow by transfusion, through the venous catheter. I held the plastic tube in my hands; I imagined I could feel the cells passing through it.

"Come on, it's your turn to work, make new blood for me, blood that will let me live for fifty more years, but don't hurt me too much." (I was thinking about the rejection reaction.)

My heart was heavy, my hands were shaking a bit, I was crying. I was alone and I wanted to stay alone for as long as the transfusion would take.

3:30 p.m.

The sun was shining, the city was colored pink and orange. They told me Diane wanted to see me. Despite the operation she had undergone only a few hours ago, she wanted to visit me and even came up four flights of stairs.

"How are you?"

"I feel as if I've fallen on my backside on a skating rink," she said, smiling.

We watched the last fifty cubic centimeters of bone marrow flow into me through the catheter. Thank you, Diane, for a wonderful lesson of courage that I will never forget, no more than I could ever forget the support given to me by Dominique, my parents, my loved ones, and the hospital staff. Thanks to the doctors who sometimes don't smile enough, but give the best treatment.

From Day 0, I was unable to leave my sterile room, and visitors had to wear a sterilized lab coat and a mask; even my food was sterilized. For five to eight weeks, I felt as if I was a fetus, protected from the outside world in a glass room.

During the first two weeks after the transplant, the effects of chemotherapy are the strongest: irritation of the mucous membranes in the mouth (mucositis) and at times of the bladder (cystitis), loss of hair, fatigue.

In my case, over a ten-day period mucositis made it impossible for me to eat. Instead, I was given nutritional supplements through the venous catheter.

To help me through a time that was very hard physically as well as emotionally, one friend had the excellent idea of bringing me labels from superior French wines and my favorite beers. I used to affix the labels to the blood or food supplement bags. Then I could sit back and watch my veins being filled with transfusions of Laffite-Rothschild, Château Latour, Hermitage, Châteauneuf-du-Pape, and company.

When I was fed with intravenous products, usually pale-colored, I would use labels from renowned white wines such as Meursault and

Puligny-Montrachet. In the morning, sometimes I would use cognac labels to jump-start the day. And in the evening, as I listened to a hockey game, I came back to my usual habit: beer!

On the fifth day, my hair began to fall out—in clumps. I had been fretting over the possibility for months, and now that it was actually happening, I found it funny—funny but inconvenient. I asked them to shave my head; why not get rid of it all if it was going to fall out anyway?

However, with a shaved head I could feel the slightest heat from the lightbulb in the bathroom ceiling and the slightest of drafts. My mother told me I looked good, like her favorite actor, Yul Brynner. Dominique told me not to worry: I had a very charming Kojak look.

"You'll see," she said, "shaved heads are in fashion."

It was that deep down, once the initial surprise was over, I didn't mind the movie-star effect; after a few days I even started to like my look.

These days, walking around with a shaved head is nothing unusual. Those who lose their hair can find some consolation; shaved heads are very fashionable when you want to be part of the artistic world or when you want to send the signal that you are alternative.

Toward the third week, my strength began to return, but my neutrophils hadn't increased. I was growing impatient. I had been cooped up in the hospital for more than a month, and my mood wasn't very good, especially in the mornings. The cognac labels weren't as funny any more!

In the fourth week, my new blood began to appear at last. But I began to run a fever, and for two weeks I had to rely on the good care of my nursing "aunts."

The hardest thing to cope with during this period was isolation. I craved news from the outside world, I wanted gossip about my classmates and my friends. I wanted to hear about everything, the funny things and the dull things. On the other hand, not all visits were captivating, and at times they helped me to appreciate my time alone.

Visitors

I had a lot of visitors, even too many, and they weren't always the people I would have preferred to see.

People have a very special attitude toward illness; their reactions can lead to astonishing behavior. Several friends I used to see on a daily basis before the transplant never came to see me even once during my hospitalization.

Any excuse is good to avoid paying a visit: "I have so much work to do these days!" "I'd love to visit you, but traffic on the bridges is terrible." "My car is in for repairs." "My girlfriend is complaining that we don't spend enough time together." One person admitted: "I'm sorry I haven't come to visit you, but I just can't stand the smell of hospitals." I answered, "That's okay; we'll call each other and have lunch next week."

In short, a sin confessed is a sin half-pardoned. These people were running away from their own fears of illness and death and, sooner or later, they will have to confront them.

What annoyed me about the many visits I did receive is that people often arrived without warning. Surprise visits could be fun, but at times, when I was tired, I had to force myself to keep up the conversation when I'd rather have been sleeping.

These intruders, these people who'd remembered I exist only since I'd fallen sick, these friends, these aunts and cousins I hadn't seen in the last ten years and who had suddenly resurfaced, I sometimes felt had come only to breathe in the little oxygen that my tiny room contained. Some forced themselves to come weekly; usually they arrived without warning, when I was sleeping, when I was washing myself using the minuscule sink at my disposal or when I was with Dominique.

As the weeks went by, conversations become more and more empty, as boring as the music piped into elevators. At first, it was fun—we'd talk about old memories, about our young days, about the funny things that had happened—but with time, conversations became one-way streets—I listened, and talked less and less. People told me the latest tabloid gossip:

"They say that Ms. X has colon cancer and they removed two feet of her intestines; but it doesn't matter, because it seems that she has twenty other feet left."

Me: "Oh, that's good."

"Such-and-such a star has gone south; her trip was ruined by gastroenteritis, she threw up and had diarrhea for a whole week."

Me: "Oh, poor her."

"Did you know that Guy Lafleur is going to have a hair transplant? They say that hurts a lot."

Me: "Oh, poor him."

After a while, they start criticizing the food in the hospital's cafeteria:

"It must be something else to eat hospital food for a whole month."

Me: "It is something else."

They talked about their little problems—a sore back, sore feet, fatigue, insomnia, trouble digesting, blah, blah, blah. Inevitably, visits ended with the usual complaints about the weather and the temperature: "They say it will be cold tomorrow. Bloody country, we'd be better off in Florida!"

I knew that these people were not ill-intentioned. I just felt like telling them that I didn't care about Ms. X's colon, the Montezuma's revenge some star suffered, or hockey star Guy Lafleur's hair. I wanted to tell them that if they found the cafeteria's broccoli mushy, they should try being fed intravenously for a whole month; they'd end up dreaming about how good it would be to eat that very same broccoli. That if the cold bothered them, they should try living in a giant test tube for sixty days; they'd fixate on a single idea: feeling the cold, energizing air on their faces.

I felt like telling them all these things, but I didn't. Because if I had, I would have hurt them, and by hurting them, I would have felt guilty. I didn't want to feel guilty. Instead, I started to restrict my visitors and to choose who they were; otherwise, I was bound to run out of patience.

Week 7: Time dragged on and on and was unbearable. I tried to relax by listening to the Rolling Stones and the Doors, by playing electronic chess, by reading mysteries. (At the time I was unaware of relaxation music or massage therapy, two things I strongly recommend today.)

I kept a diary, to express my frustration and anxieties and to make sure I would remember the good things about my hospitalization: the appearance of new blood cells, visits from people I love, or simply a sunrise over the refineries in Montreal's East End.

I also had to confront and live with fear, the fear of transplant rejection, the fear of infection, the fear of falling ill once again, the fear of death.

Sometimes I was pleasantly surprised; for example, one evening Serge came to listen to the hockey game with me. He smuggled in two bottles of cold beer under his coat and we drank them clandestinely!

Family and friends were a great comfort. And another great comfort was the very precious help of another transplant recipient. Yves, a native of the Lac Saint-Jean region, underwent the same procedure twelve months before I did for a different sort of illness. It was not so much his account of his ordeal that encouraged me as the fact that I saw him alive, that I heard him talking about his girlfriend, his upcoming engagement, and his newfound passion: birds. His living testimonial was irreplaceable.

The Quiver of Life

During this time, I learned how valuable life is. Each evening, stretched out on my bed, eyes closed, I saw very far. I traveled to the sky and the stars, to beautiful landscapes, to the sea, its islands and its shores, to the forest, its colors and its smells. I listened to my heartbeat, until it reached my ears, and I quivered, I quivered from the tips of my fingers to the tips of my toes, and the quivers traveled through my body, up to my head.

I called the feeling "the quiver of life." It contributed to my healing and will stay with me for a long time to come.

The Period Following Hospitalization

Going Home

Going home is like cutting the umbilical cord. The intravenous catheter is removed, you are given lengthy advice and surgical masks to wear into the fourth month after the transplant, an appointment is made with the outpatient clinic, and you are sent home.

"At last," I told myself on that December 21. "Goodbye solutes, transfusion pumps, blood tests, masked visitors, and limited space. Hello french fries and steak, beer, chips, friends, and hockey. Hello kissing and cuddling with Dominique. I'm back to life again."

But suddenly the fear of viruses, bacteria, the cold, and pollution robs you of all your self-assurance. You're not as eager to leave the comfortable nest that the hospital now seems to be. This reaction can easily be compared to the separation anxiety found in children who refuse to stray too far from their mothers.

When I left the security of the hospital environment, I experienced fear and anxiety. This is a normal and natural feeling, and all patients who have undergone a lengthy hospitalization face this particular stumbling block. Yet when patients leave the hospital, their immune systems have all the tools they need to fight infections.

My Second Life

The temperature was a few degrees below zero and it was snowing. Behind the house there was a skating rink, like the ones that used to dot every neighborhood before the politicians began to cut budgets.

On the skating rink I could see children—very healthy children, believe me. Hats, mittens, long scarves, three sweaters, nothing could stop them: they skated fast, they turned on a dime, the ice crunched

39

under their blades. With red cheeks and frost-tipped hair, they squealed and laughed!

I put on my skates, a warm coat, and my mask to protect me against germs, and I hopped onto the ice. After thirty minutes I was out of breath, coughing, and every bone in my body hurts. But oh! how very happy I was!

One kid asked: "Mister, why are you wearing a mask?"

In five seconds flat the whole troop was around me; they had all noticed but had been pretending not to.

"I had a serious disease, I just got out of the hospital. I have to wear this mask so I don't catch any germs."

"Which disease?" asked a boy knee-high to a grasshopper, with eyes like saucers.

"Leukemia."

"Terry Fox's disease?" asked an older kid. Terry Fox had just died and his exploits had made him a national hero, an ideal for all young people, and for me.

Another kid answered, "No, Terry Fox's disease was cancer of the legs."

"Is leukemia more serious than cancer of the legs?" the first kid asked before I had a chance to answer his initial question.

"Both diseases are very serious; leukemia is blood cancer and Terry Fox had bone cancer that began in his leg."

"That's why they cut off his leg," said a small, bright-eyed girl who played hockey remarkably well.

"Do you have hair?" another kid wanted to know.

"Not much, but look, it's growing back," I said, removing my hat to show them a thin layer of down.

"You must be cold," said the girl.

"Yes, it's not very warm for my head! So why don't we continue with our game?"

Thus I spent the first two hours of my convalescence.

The Fourth Month and Beyond

At last I banished the mask against germs and resumed my education; but perhaps I did so a bit too quickly, because the following months were punctuated with complications.

A chronic rejection (chronic GVH), with effects on the liver and tear and saliva glands, forced me to take high doses of cortisone over an eighteen-month period. Subsequently, the doses were reduced and the cells stopped attacking the organs. A viral infection of the skin, commonly known as shingles, forced me to return to the hospital for another two-week stay, much to my displeasure.

As I look back, I now realize that six months of convalescence should be the minimum before resuming normal activities.

After the second year, I had all of my strength back, I was no longer taking any form of medication, and I was living perfectly normally, just as I was before the transplant.

As you can see, the war isn't over immediately after the transplant. The first year can be hard for patients with chronic GVH. They complain of a dry mouth and dry eyes, and they notice that their hair isn't growing back as quickly as they had expected. Some suffer side effects from antirejection medication, including a swelling of the face and increased pilosity.

But in most cases, rejection diminishes gradually; over time, medication doses decrease as well and, consequently, so do side effects. Among other things, GVH has the precious quality of diminishing the risk of a relapse because of its "antileukemia transplant" (graft vs. leukemia) effect; in other words, it provides protection against a repeated bout of leukemia.

Am I truly cured? Will the disease come back?

Even after several years, these questions still arise. Of course, my confidence is building, but worries still survive deep down inside. That doesn't matter. What does matter is tackling problems one by one, living one day at a time, and staying hopeful. This is a lesson illness has taught me, as it has taught me to reflect on death. Only a few years ago, I never would have dared to bring up the subject. Like everyone else, I preferred to avoid it; after all, death is something that is upsetting to everyone. Yet, we must discuss death. We must be aware that it is the normal outcome of our existence, a stage that is common to all of us as living beings.

Among some species, the life cycle is very simple and very brief. Such is not the case with human beings. Our life cycle is complex and unpredictable, subject to the laws of fate, of wealth and poverty, often dependent on the social and political nature of our native country, linked to the fragile equilibrium between our defense mechanisms and our ability to adapt.

For example, over the past forty years more damage has been done to our environment than in the past twenty centuries. Factors that have an aggressive effect on our bodies—pollution, radiation, new chemical substances—are more and more numerous and our bodies are unable to adjust quickly enough; the result is illnesses that can be fatal.

But whether it happens unexpectedly as the result of an accident or whether it comes about because of a serious illness, death is merely the continuation of life, a passage to another life. People who have lived through near-death experiences, such as cardiac arrest, describe this passage as a long tunnel with a strong and bright light at its end. As the light draws nearer, it relieves anxiety and fear, creating a feeling of great interior serenity.

If that is truly death, I hope that each of us can experience the passage to light and serenity.

Years Later

Reflections on Health

Even before I contracted leukemia, social problems, the environment, and health problems were of concern to me; but illness truly confirmed my convictions with regard to these issues. And today, I feel that we live too much as spectators; because problems are presented to us with a great deal of complexity, we end up believing that only politicians and experts can solve them.

These same politicians waste our funds on arms, trips, and receptions while everywhere patients are crowded into emergency ward corridors, while children are poisoned with heavy metals, while we drink PCBs and all manner of toxins in our tap water, in parts per million said to be acceptable for our health. And what of the developing world, where every twenty minutes a child dies due to lack of food and basic care? In the meantime, funds devoted to research, social services, the environment, and foreign aid are repeatedly cut.

What to do? How and where to begin?

First of all, be well informed. We may not be able to keep abreast of all issues at once, but we can focus our efforts on one issue that is of particular interest to us. Second, do not be afraid to express your opinions, to take a stand. Finally, take concrete action, on your own scale.

For example, responding to a survey is a good way to express your opinion on a topic and to have some degree of influence on decision makers, especially since our current politicians have a strong tendency to lead through poll results. Unfortunately, they also have a tendency to be shortsighted. As they strive to solve today's problems as quickly and as economically as possible, they sometimes forget that they must leave a legacy to future generations. We are all involved in the choices to be made.

Too often, human beings tend to amass wealth without thinking of the long-term consequences. We even go so far as to proclaim this tiny planet as our own, when we are merely one type of living being among many others on Earth. Our quest for instant happiness must not jeopardize the future and the survival of this planet.

But then again, what is happiness?

For me, happiness can be sitting by the front door, looking at the sidewalk below and the people strolling by on it. It is the smell of a recently mown lawn, of trees after a quenching rain, of new foliage. It is the elderly man who gets just as much enjoyment from walking his dog as he does from feeding the pigeons and the squirrels in the park. It is the wonderment of life. For me, true happiness is hidden in a host of small, day-to-day things that we often forget to see and experience.

Our Attitude toward Illness

My adventure—during which, from one day to the next, I was forced to face a serious illness, its often difficult treatment, and the fear that in the end the outcome would be negative—made me aware that health is very fragile, that it should be protected at all times, and that we must not wait for illness to occur before we take care of it.

In addition to the many forms of exterior aggression I have referred to, such as pollution, radiation, infection, and the accidents that fate puts in our path, some well-known aggressors come from within us. For example, there are our reactions to stress and states of depression, anxiety, and anguish. These inner conflicts can diminish our desire to be healthy and lead us, unconsciously, to fall into the cycle of illness.

The attitude we have toward our life determines its quality and duration. Thus, people who love life, who have the will to live problem-free until age one hundred, can reach beyond their limitations when illness strikes them. These are the people who defy the statistics of the so-called survival rate or life expectancy linked to particular illnesses. These are the people we refer to when we speak of spontaneous remission, the type of healing that science is unable to explain.

The Patient and the Health Care System

Unfortunately, in the labyrinth of modern medicine, where diagnostic and therapeutic methods are developed at high-tech speed, it is not uncommon for patients to feel completely overwhelmed by the events surrounding their illness; in spite of themselves, they feel dependent on a system that they do not understand.

During my hospitalization, I missed the presence of doctors. I felt that they did not come to see me often enough, and when they did come, they were always in a rush. Many patients and their families feel this same lack of attention and they accuse doctors of not providing them with enough information. Today, now that I myself am a doctor, I have a better understanding of the situation. The medical infrastructure, in all leading-edge areas such as bone marrow transplants, requires doctors to double as administrators, to manage budgets that are consistently cut from year to year. They also must contribute to research programs and publish a certain number of scientific articles, read up on the latest developments, and take part in conventions to keep pace and to be in a position to offer the best possible treatment to patients. On a daily basis, they act as teachers who train medical students, and when they are on call, they are responsible for all of the hospital's emergency cases. When the time comes to visit hospitalized patients, they review files, discuss matters with the nurses, and concentrate on those patients who are most seriously ill or who are experiencing complications.

In short, the way in which a doctor's time is structured leaves no opportunity to sit and discuss events with patients whose illnesses are evolving positively. Often, patients tell me that because they have barely seen their doctor throughout their stay in the hospital, they feel like numbers. In such instances, I reply that with this particular type of illness, not being visited by their doctor very often is a good sign, a sign that things are going well.

Having suffered from an illness that was described as incurable, I can assure you that it's not important to have hypersensitive doctors holding your hand. What is important is having the best doctors, capable of taking care of you effectively and efficiently.

However, despite the development of super-specializations, health care professionals must also maintain a balance between science and the caregiving relationship with the patient. At all times, they must keep in mind that patients and their families are going through a time of suffering, dependence, and anxiety, that an understanding of the illness and of diagnostic methods leads to active participation in a treatment program and facilitates the building of trust with the treatment team. In turn, this climate of understanding and trust reinforces a positive attitude in the face of the illness and makes it easier to tolerate treatments and, in the end, to heal.

In this world of high technology, reconciling illness with science is the most fascinating and exciting of all challenges facing the medical community.

The Present

Today, I can assert that life is fascinating.

People often ask me, "Did illness change your life?" Surely, but in what way? To find out, I would have had to clone another Robert who would have lived through the last seventeen years without an illness, a type of placebo with whom I could compare myself. I don't know where my clone would be at this point, but I know where I am.

Several thousand days have gone by since the miraculous transplant. Health is something I once again take for granted; I am in better shape than most people my age, I exercise, I eat well, and I keep excesses to a minimum. What a joy it is to be healthy! Even if ghosts sometimes emerge, I know that I am cured and that I will live to be an old man.

After my transplant, I finished medical school, worked as a general practitioner for one year in an outlying region, then went back to school to become a hematologist-oncologist. I dreamt of becoming a specialist to heal cancer-stricken patients, but for two reasons my dream never came true.

The first reason is that studies in a medical specialty are extremely demanding and laborious; for the first seven years, specialists have no control over their work schedules and must be on call for a full day several times per month. Living at this pace is feasible when you've never been sick; however, in my case, before each twenty-four-hour on-call period, my thirst for freedom was so strong that I would become anxious and ill-tempered.

The second reason I discovered during my two-month oncology internship: I was so taken with cancer patients that I would visit them in the evening and on my days off. I spent long hours talking with their families, and during this time I set up the Bone Marrow Transplant Foundation, a nonprofit organization that assists patients and subsidizes research.

This was a wonderful time, but it was exhausting both for Dominique and for myself. I wasn't home very often, and when I did come in late at night, I was tired, irritable, and day-to-day problems seemed completely unimportant to me. One day, one of my bosses told me, "You know, Robert, just because you're fighting a war, you don't have to be a general." So I left the specialty, realizing that sooner or later my excessive empathy would lead me to total exhaustion. I decided to work as an emergency ward and critical care doctor, and I have no regrets that I made that choice.

Our Destiny

Throughout our lives, we must face situations that are more or less predictable and, at times, uncontrollable. From childhood to death, we must make choices and decisions that demand effort and that sometimes cause suffering.

There are many ordinary aggressors. Illnesses, accidents, physical and psychological assaults, emotional pain, loneliness, routine, and hard work are only a few examples. In the face of these various situations, we can let ourselves go, we can focus on our misfortune, we can drag with us an unhappy or miserable childhood, we can rebel against our parents and our family, and, throughout a lifetime, we can be unhappy.

The alternative attitude is much more demanding; it consists of confronting fate with strength and courage. For some people, psychotherapy leads to a better understanding of the past and the ability to grow.

Sometimes, under other circumstances, it is best to flee and, in doing so, avoid the kind of uncontrollable situations that can damage our emotional and physical health.

Henri Laborit has written a very interesting book on the subject, in which, in light of biological discoveries, he questions the role of our free will, of our very personality, in the way we confront aggressors. "Rebelling," he says, "is heading for ruin, because a rebellion, if it is carried out in a group, immediately creates a hierarchical scale of submission within that same group, and rebellion in and of itself leads to the rebel's submission.... All that remains is flight."

In short, the way each person faces difficult situations is intimately linked to his or her personality. However, too often people underestimate their ability to confront life's tragedies. Always running from problems leads us nowhere, because doing so deprives us of the rich experiences that success or failure bring with them. On the other hand, as Henri Laborit explains, we should not live in a constant state of rebellion, because this places us in a context of submission that, in the long run, is every bit as harmful to our physical and psychological well-being. Each day, we must strike the right balance between an attitude of confrontation and an attitude of flight from trials.

Albert Einstein had very little faith in the haphazard; he claimed that everything was predictable and calculable. In the strictly mathematical sense, this is true. Increasingly, science is decoding nature's secrets—secrets that formerly were attributed to the haphazard, to the will of God, even to the devil. Barely ten years ago, we used to say that the mentally ill, and schizophrenics in particular, were possessed by demonic spirits; we used to say that it was impossible to choose a baby's gender. Today, we know that schizophrenia is caused by a defective gene and that laboratory procedures can make it possible to choose a child's gender before the mother's egg is fertilized.

A psychiatrist friend once told me that one of the main causes of traffic accidents is a lack of concentration on the part of one of the drivers involved. In fact, we have all experienced situations in which our concentration was affected by job-related stress or by a state of depression. An argument with a colleague, spouse, or child, a host of causes other than drugs or alcohol, can diminish our concentration on the road and can increase the risk of having an accident. Yet most often, we accuse fate or destiny.

So we have several mechanisms through which we can influence the seemingly haphazard situations that fate places in our path, to avoid catastrophes and to attract positive occurrences, and consequently to live a happier and healthier life.

There is nothing new in the statement that several illnesses are directly related to habits over which we have full control. By eating healthy, by exercising, by adopting a sound lifestyle, and by limiting any form of excess, we live well and we live longer.

I could give you dozens of examples of people who have recovered from serious illnesses and who have continued to practice harmful habits. Stricken with lung cancer, leukemia, or serious heart disease, as an excuse or a justification these people who have been very close to death and who have kept their bad habits, smoking in particular, often say, "You know, Doctor, the only thing I have left are cigarettes. They are my only pleasure." Or they tell me, "Smoking helps me control my stress." Or perhaps, "Dying of heart disease or dying of cancer, what difference does it make? I don't want to grow old, I don't want to die in a home." In essence, these people seek a magical cure, one that will require minimal personal effort.

Studies have shown that people in poor overall condition (the obese, smokers, the sedentary, and the stressed) are also those who early in their lives suffered from chronic illnesses (heart disease, chronic bronchitis, emphysema, diabetes, etc.) and who, for dozens of years, have had a very poor quality of life because of repeated hospitalization and the need to submit to tests that can be painful and unpleasant. Often they must move to group homes before they die.

Healthy individuals live much longer and enjoy an excellent quality of life until the day they contract a serious illness that leads to a quick death. Living a healthy and long life is the future built by people who take good care of themselves.

We have an important role to play in how our fate unfolds. It is easy to place ourselves in situations that are a major risk for our health and that may even put our lives in jeopardy. So we have to learn to avoid mistakes and wait for opportunities, to think before taking action, and to act moderately. This process is what we refer to as wisdom.

Death

Death frightens me. And so I want to die at age ninety, suddenly, on my sailboat, in a foggy harbor, with a woman, while we are making love. Why not? I loathe death; I want to do all I can to keep it away from myself and from my family, my friends, and my patients.

Whether I see it in television reports, in newspaper articles, or in an emergency ward, death always has an enormous effect on me. Sadly, our society, particularly the young, have become desensitized to violence, to tragedy, and to death. To a great extent, this modern-day phenomenon is closely linked to the media, which constantly look for ways to increase ratings by promoting the sensational. Over time, human beings have become less sensitive to violence and death; our tolerance toward what is unacceptable has increased steadily and without our realizing it. In our daily lives, we carry the burden of gratuitous violence.

Insensitivity to death is common in the hospital environment. In ten years, I have seen dozens of elderly people dying alone in the far reaches of hospitals. I have also seen anonymous heroes, health care workers, or volunteers willing to accompany the elderly in this, the last stage of their lives.

I remember an old man who arrived by ambulance because of a sudden paralysis in his right side. His hygiene was terrible and he was in a lamentable state. The ambulance attendant said, "You should have seen his apartment, Doctor—a complete mess. The neighbors called us because no one had seen the man in over three days. We don't know much about him; all we have is his son's telephone number. We've notified him; he should be coming in."

After a thorough examination and diagnostic tests, we concluded that the eighty-three-year-old patient was suffering from three very serious problems: a stroke, a myocardial infarction, and pneumonia. Despite medical treatment, the situation deteriorated quickly and his chances of surviving were slim.

Since we had no news of his son, I decided to call him. "Sir, I am Dr. Patenaude and I would like to notify you that your father is very ill. He has had a stroke and a heart attack and he has pneumonia. He is in the emergency ward right now, he is extremely weak, and I am not sure that he will survive."

"Is he conscious?" asked the son.

"I don't know; his right side is paralyzed because of the stroke. He is asleep, but he isn't in any pain."

"So if he isn't conscious, what good will it do to come to the hospital?" And then the man added, "How long do you think he will live?"

"I don't know—a few hours at most."

"In that case," said the son, "call me back when it's over. I'll drop by to pick up his belongings and sign the papers."

I had the old man placed in a small room off the emergency ward. André, an attendant, cleaned him and even took the time to shave his beard. I went on to other patients and André decided to use his lunch hour to stay with the man. He held his hand, talking softly about all sorts of things—his own family, his children, his twenty-five years working in the emergency ward, his latest fishing trip. The old man passed away peacefully and with dignity. Then André resumed his day, with no expectation of a medal or an award for his gesture.

Another anonymous hero died more recently: my father. All his life, he worked hard for his family. I was brought up on the South Shore of Montreal, but my father never wanted to fit into the suburban mold. He didn't earn very much and he refused to waste his money on new cars, bought every three years to impress the neighbors, or on the fight against weeds and dandelions in hopes of earning the "Mr. South Shore Lawn" title.

No, my father was not like the other fathers in the neighborhood. Every weekend we went to the country to go camping, and at least once each summer he brought us to the seashore. My sisters and I were keenly aware of nature and travel at a very young age. Family life in the outdoors is simple and healthy. For children, the day-to-day discoveries that nature holds are inestimable chances to learn—lessons that last a lifetime. I still remember the first frog I captured, and the first fish I caught when I was five years old. I also remember being scolded for killing a sparrow with a BB gun.

At the age of forty-eight, my father was diagnosed with a grave heart disease. He underwent surgery, but unfortunately there were serious complications and, as a result, he suffered permanent damage to his kidneys and his mental capabilities. That he suffered from a heart ailment came as no surprise to us—his heart was precisely what was greatest and most fragile about him. His quality of life was heavily affected: he would run out of breath at the slightest effort, his legs would swell, and most importantly, his mental faculties were diminished.

Eventually, he lost his job, his house, and his car. The last ten years of his life he owed to my mother, who took care of him until the end. Despite her night job in a restaurant, she never considered placing him in a home.

My father left us at the age of fifty-eight, on November 8, 1992, the same day I was celebrating the tenth anniversary of my bone marrow transplant. He died with his family at his side, in a calm and restful way.

I was on call in the emergency ward that night. At around one o'clock in the morning my mother telephoned me to tell me that my father had been taken to the Cardiology Institute. For the fourth time in six months, his lungs were filled with liquid; his heart was very weak. Despite increasingly strong doses, his medication no longer seemed to be working. Given the situation, the doctor suggested that the family come to his bedside.

I called my friend Serge, asked him to replace me, and went to join my family. On that autumn night, I wrote the following:

> There are moments in a life that shatter time and, subsequently, that stay with us forever. My father, lying on a hospital bed, breathing with obvious difficulty. This time the medication for his heart and kidneys was having no effect, his illness had progressed too far. Around three o'clock in the morning, he fell asleep, finding relief with a dose of morphine. Then there came a time when the breaths he was taking were longer and longer. We were at his side and we watched as he stopped breathing completely.

My mother bent to kiss him. Then my father sighed three times, as if saying, "I love you. Thank you for these thirty-five wonderful years of love, thank you for your strength, thank you for your courage." My parents had always loved each other as they had when they first met.

His heart stopped beating, and then there was nothing, not a sound, as if the ocean had come to a standstill, no more breathing, as if the wind had stopped blowing in the trees. We cried.

Later, we went into a small room where a nurse kindly gave us coffee. The chaplain came to us and offered the following words of comfort: "His heart and his body are gone, but don't be sad. His soul will always be with you."

This is how my father died.

Today, when we are with his grandchildren, we often talk about my father, always with a great deal of pride, often with laughter.

When we see a beautiful landscape: "Oh, if Dad could see this."

Or jokingly: "Remember the time Dad fell into the water? Did we have a good time laughing at him!" When we take his grandchildren on outdoor activities: "You see, this fishing technique is one that your grandfather taught me." Today, as the chaplain told us, our father is with us and everything he taught us is passed on.

Very recently, I was forced to face death once again: the death of my sister Diane. Diane, who had been my transplant donor, whose blood cells are still alive in my body.

Diane was a schizophrenic. But for ten years, her illness was stable and we were astounded to learn of her death one September evening. Without warning, she had thrown herself into the emptiness, from Jacques Cartier Bridge. Her inner suffering must have been unbearable. As I write these lines, I still have a hard time believing that she is dead. I have a hard time accepting her death. And I still don't understand why my sister didn't reach out for my help. It is so frustrating to feel so powerless in the face of fate. But above all, I refuse to judge her actions.

In Conclusion...

I am in the best health I have ever been in. I run five miles to the top of Mount Saint Hilaire several times a week, I regularly go biking, and I go sailing as often as I can. My sailboat is my sanctuary: no pager, no telephone, no television, only the peace and quiet of family life, the perfect balance between the forces of nature, machine, and human being.

I often think of the many transplant recipients I have known and those who, sadly, did not survive. Of the first thirty bone marrow transplant recipients, only ten are still alive. I want to express my recognition to all of those who are no longer with us and who have left behind wonderful memories and a magnificent lesson in courage.

Thank you to the pioneers in the fight against cancer (patients, researchers, medical personnel) who have contributed to the improvement of treatments. Today, we save 70 percent of leukemic children treated with chemotherapy and adults who receive a bone marrow transplant. Thank you to Dr. Thomas for his wonderful research on leukemia, research that gave me a second chance at life and for which he received the 1990 Nobel prize for medicine. Thank you to my doctor and friend Dr. Perreault, now chief of one of the most successful research centers in Canada, who works in the field of immunology.

The experience of illness, of fear, of suffering and, in the end, of healing, has shown me that only we can make the decision to shy away, to stay put, or to move forward as events unfold. Throughout our entire lifetimes, we search for love, for our dreams and our ideals.

As we move forward over time, we begin to feel pride, to feel that we have grown and, on a starry night late in the month of August, that we can reach up and graze the stars with our fingertips.

> And when you want something, the entire universe conspires to give
> you means to make your wish come true.
>
> The Alchemist

One day, cancer will be nothing more than a bad memory.

The Cell

The cell is the smallest living structure in our bodies. When several cells with the same very specific function are grouped together, they form an organ. The liver, lungs, brain, heart, muscles, bone marrow, and all other organs in our bodies are composed of cells. When referring to blood, we use the term *blood cell*.

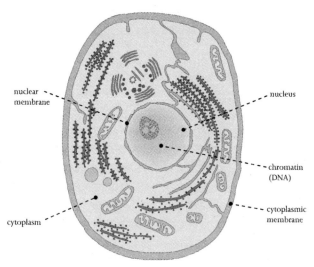

nuclear membrane

nucleus

chromatin (DNA)

cytoplasmic membrane

cytoplasm

The cell

The membrane serves as the cell's barrier. It is semipermeable; in other words, certain substances can permeate it, while others cannot. It is also very flexible, which allows the cell to take on a limitless number of shapes. Thanks to these two characteristics, the cell can accomplish a multitude of tasks.

The cytoplasm is the region located between the nucleus and the membrane. All products needed to ensure that the cell functions properly (for example, hemoglobin, antibodies, enzymes, proteins) are manufactured in the cytoplasm; this is also where the cell digests the bacteria it eats.

In some ways, the nucleus is the cell's brain. A long chain referred to as DNA is found in the nucleus. This chain contains all of the genetic information needed for a cell's multiplication and functioning. When the cell divides, the DNA chain breaks down into rods referred to as chromosomes. Recent studies lead scientists to believe that an anomaly in the DNA is at the root of the unnatural behavior of the cancerous cell, which multiplies repeatedly.

Blood

See Color Plate No. 1.

Blood is to humans what sap is to a tree: a living liquid that brings energy to all of our organs.

Since time began, blood has been a source of inspiration for poets and writers; since time began, it has sparked enormous curiosity among researchers. The former claim that, throughout our lifetimes, blood carries through our veins the happy memories of our childhood, the folly of our adolescence, and the grand passions that mark our adulthood. The latter study it, analyze it, and attempt to find the key to its smallest secrets. Like voyeurs, behind their microscopes they admire the shapes of its blood cells, bathed in the gold of polarizing light and spread out on spotless glass slides.

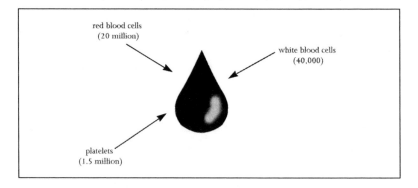

red blood cells
(20 million)

white blood cells
(40,000)

platelets
(1.5 million)

The cells contained in one drop of blood

Our internal organs, such as the lungs, liver, and kidneys, are immobile; while blood is liquid and while it travels throughout the body, it should be considered an organ as well.

Blood is composed of two phases: a liquid phase, plasma, and a solid phase, cells.

There are three types of cells: red, white, and platelets. All three float in the plasma. These cells are so small that it would be possible to line up more than one hundred red cells on the head of a pin. In a single drop of blood, there are more than twenty million red cells, forty thousand white cells, and one and a half million platelets. Imagine the total number of cells contained in five liters of human blood!

In laboratories, it is easy to separate blood cells and plasma, using a technique called centrifugation.

Plasma

Plasma is a citrin liquid used as a support mechanism for millions of cells that are suspended in it. However, it is more than a carrier; it also contains a number of products that ensure the proper functioning of our bodies, such as glucose, minerals (calcium, sodium, potassium, chlorine, etc.), proteins (albumin, antibodies, proteins needed for blood coagulation, etc.), soluble fats (cholesterol, triglycerides), and a number of products resulting from organ activity (urea, lactic acid, creatine, etc.).

Types of Blood Cells

In the illustration below the cells seem large; in reality, they are minuscule.

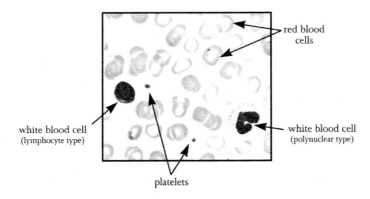

red blood cells

white blood cell (lymphocyte type)

white blood cell (polynuclear type)

platelets

Red Blood Cells

Red blood cells look like small sacs with a flat center; they have no nucleus and their main role is to transport hemoglobin, which in turn transports the oxygen picked up from the lungs.

As they travel through the arteries, red blood cells distribute oxygen to all of the organs in our body (brain, heart, muscles, etc.). At the same time, they pick up the carbon dioxide (CO_2) from these organs and, through the veins, transport it to the lungs.

When red blood cells are filled with oxygen, they are bright red. When they are transporting carbon dioxide they are a bluish color. This explains the bright red color of arterial blood and the bluish color of venous blood (see "The Cardiorespiratory System," pages 68–69). There are a very high number of red blood cells: approximately five million per cubic millimeter of blood; their average lifespan is 120 days. They are manufactured mainly in bone marrow.

If their number decreases or if the quantity of hemoglobin they carry decreases, the resulting condition is known as anemia. Anemia has several causes, the most common being loss of blood (heavy menstruation, giving birth, intestinal bleeding, or a secondary hemorrhage due to a wound); it can also be caused by a lack of iron or vitamins (folic acid and vitamin B_{12}). In some instances, anemia can be the warning sign of more serious illnesses that decrease the number of red blood cells the body produces: certain cases of aplasia, leukemia, and lymphoma.

On their surface, red blood cells carry the antigens of the ABO and Rh blood types.

White Blood Cells

White cells are true cells: they have a nucleus, an intracellular space (cytoplasm), and a membrane.

The nucleus can have several shapes; for example, it can be round and formed of a single lobe, or it can have several lobes and appear to be multiple. The intracellular space (cytoplasm) contains enzymes, substances used to digest foreign bodies. The membrane carries the HLA tissue groups; HLAs (H for human, L for leucocytes, and A for antigens) are groups that define each human being, and their role is vital in the transplant rejection reaction.

There are two large families of white cells: lymphocytes and myelocytes. These two classes of white cells are differentiated by their nucleus and the color of their intracellular space (see Color Plate No. 1).

Myelocytes

This class accounts for 55 to 65 percent of all white cells.

Early researchers believed that these cells had several nuclei, which is why they referred to them as "polynuclears." Today, we know that these cells have only one nucleus, composed of several lobes that are linked together by a system of fine threads.

The intracellular space contains small grains (granules) that pick up colorants and take on bluish or reddish tints. These granules are what give these corpuscles their alternate name: granulocytes. The color of grains can differentiate neutrophilic (slightly bluish) polynuclears, eosinophilic (red) polynuclears, and basophilic (very bluish) polynuclears.

Polynuclears have several functions:

- Neutrophilic polynuclears, specialized in bacteria phagocytosis (digestion), play an important role in the anti-infection battle. Their number increases when infections are present.
- Eosinophilic polynuclears play a role in allergic reactions and in the body's defense against parasites.
- As for basophilic polynuclears, their role is unknown.

The terms *granulocytes* and *polynuclears* are accurate, and both commonly used to designate the myelocytes "families."

Lymphocytes

Lymphocytes make up the remaining 35 to 45 percent of white blood cells. They have a large, oval nucleus, but no grains. These blood cells are manufactured mainly by the lymph nodes.

Because they are specialized in the manufacture of antibodies, lymphocytes play an important part in the fight against infections and transplant rejections. Antibodies attack viruses, bacteria, and foreign bodies.

Lymphocytes can also "remember" some viruses, preventing subsequent infections. This phenomenon is known as immunization.

Platelets

Platelets look like minuscule sacs and have the property of sticking to one another to form a blood clot. Blood clots seal off the walls of veins and arteries, which prevents bleeding (hemorrhages). When the number of platelets decreases, the patient is more susceptible to bruises and hemorrhages.

Bone Marrow
See Color Plate No. 2.

Bone marrow constitutes the major industrial center in our bodies—it has the major task of manufacturing blood. In fact, it replaces all of our blood once every twenty days.

This change is progressive: each second, bone marrow produces more than ten million blood cells, which flow into the blood. At the same time, ten million other blood cells die; thus, equilibrium exists at all times.

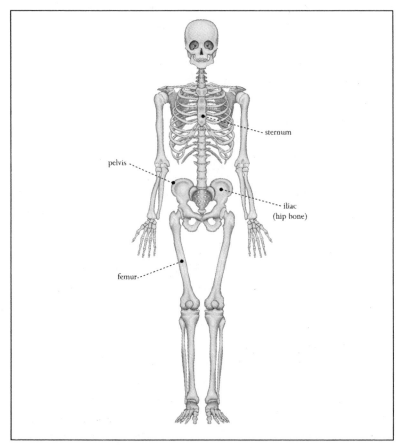

The bones in our bodies containing marrow rich in stem cells

Bone marrow works according to very precise rules; it adjusts to the rules of supply and demand by increasing or decreasing its production. It adapts quickly to all of the conditions that can prevail in our bodies; when an infection is present, it produces more white blood cells so that the body is better equipped to fight germs. Once the infection is under control, the number of white blood cells produced drops to its normal level. In situations where there is hemorrhaging, the production of red blood cells increases until their number returns to its normal level.

Bone marrow also reacts to certain natural phenomena; for example, at high altitudes, where oxygen is less plentiful, bone marrow manufactures more red blood cells, which results in better oxygenation of the body's organs. Athletes who are aware of this process often train at high altitudes a few weeks before competing. When they return to sea level, they benefit from better muscle oxygenation and their performance levels are higher.

Bone marrow has a liquid consistency and is found in the center of all of the bones in the body. It contains stem cells (cells with the ability to multiply and to produce blood cells), which it uses to renew our blood supply throughout our lifetimes. We call this the hemopoietic system (see pages 67–68). The stem cells can move into the blood stream by using the hormone named colony stimulating factor.

The bone marrow found in the sternum and hip bone contains the highest number of stem cells. This is where doctors do bone marrow puncture and bone marrow biopsies. These two tests are essential to arrive at a diagnosis (see Chapter 3).

Blood Clot Formation

We could not survive without the presence of mechanisms through which our bodies seal the breaks in our arteries and our veins—at all times, we are exposed to accidents (traumas, cuts, fractures) that can lead to lesions in our blood vessels. Without the formation of blood clots, these lesions would cause an uncontrollable loss of blood that would quickly jeopardize our lives. Several malignant blood diseases weaken the body's ability to form blood clots.

Hemorrhages can be external (breaks in vessels located in the skin) or internal (breaks in vessels located inside certain organs, such as the stomach, intestine, kidney, and brain). Minor hemorrhages are quickly brought under control through the formation of a blood clot, but serious hemorrhages sometimes require surgical intervention; if, for example, a large blood vessel is torn, a stitch is needed to bring the two vessel walls together, which stops the bleeding.

The formation of a blood clot is also called blood coagulation or hemostasis. It requires the presence of platelets and substances known as coagulation factors that are found in blood plasma. Numbers are assigned to each of these factors. Coagulation factors react to one another in a sequential series and form a trellis that incorporates platelets: a blood clot.

The Causes of Increased Bleeding

Usually, blood clots form quickly and all minor bleeding stops within a few minutes. But several causes can slow the formation of a blood clot; in addition to a decrease in the number of platelets, referred to previously, some forms of medication, some illnesses, and a vitamin deficiency sometimes slow down the process leading to blood clot formation, thus increasing the risk of severe hemorrhage.

Medications that Delay the Formation of Blood Clots

The most common medication known to have an effect on coagulation is aspirin. Aspirin decreases the efficiency of platelets, which slows the formation of blood clots. The effect of aspirin can last for more than two weeks following the ingestion of a single tablet.

Anti-inflammatories and antibiotics can also have a negative effect on coagulation.

Because they can result in severe hemorrhaging, medications that decrease the efficiency of platelets should never be used by patients under treatment for malignant blood diseases without prior consultation with a physician.

Other medications (such as warfarin) are intentionally used to slow the formation of blood clots, or to "thin the blood," as some patients say. These anticoagulants are used to treat patients who have artificial heart valves or who have suffered from phlebitis or pulmonary embolisms in the past.

Diseases that Slow the Formation of Blood Clots

Among congenital diseases (see "Congenital Diseases of the Blood System" in Chapter 4) that affect coagulation factors and slow the formation of blood clots, the most common are Type A hemophilia and Type B hemophilia.

Severe liver diseases decrease the formation of coagulation factors and increase the risk of severe hemorrhage.

All malignant blood diseases and all kidney diseases lead to renal failure. Serious infections and certain inflammatory diseases can affect the formation of blood clots.

Vitamin Deficiencies

Due either to malnutrition or to poor digestive absorption, vitamin deficiencies can increase bleeding.

Vitamin K is crucial to the formation of II, VII, IX, and X blood coagulation factors; a lack of vitamin K leads to a decrease in these factors, which slows down the chain reaction leading to the formation of a blood clot.

Deficiencies in vitamin C, vitamin B_{12}, and folic acid can lead to increased bleeding.

Symptoms Suggesting Coagulation Problems

The appearance of small red dots (petechia) or larger blotches (purpura and bruises) on the skin often indicates problems that can be traced to platelets. Bleeding in the stomach or in other regions of the intestine and bleeding within joints (hemarthrosis) is more likely linked to a problem with coagulation factors.

Some types of bleeding are perfectly normal among people in good health; for example, menstruation or the type of bleeding associated with superficial cuts. But any increase in the duration or the quantity of such bleeding should be discussed with a physician, who will decide whether to evaluate blood clot formation. Evaluating coagulation factors and platelets is part of the basic blood testing procedure.

Blood and the Body's Main Systems

Blood, a vital liquid essential to all of our organs, carries the nutrients and oxygen our bodies need. It also plays a role in eliminating waste, since it carries toxic materials to the organs that excrete them from the body.

The study of anatomy and the functioning of the human body is very complex. To facilitate it, using illustrations, we will examine each of the main organs, grouped into individual systems. We will look at the hemopoietic system, the cardiorespiratory system, the central nervous system, the digestive system, and the urinary system. These systems do not constitute all of the human body's anatomy, but they are closely linked to blood and, consequently, they are often affected by malignant blood diseases.

The Hemopoietic System

The hemopoietic system groups together bone marrow, the spleen, and lymph nodes, which are all linked by small vessels knows as lymphatic ducts.

Lymph Node System

Lymph nodes are the organs in which white lymphocyte-type blood cells multiply; their function is to fight infections. Lymph nodes increase in volume as a reaction to certain cancers, infections, or inflammatory diseases. We call this lymphadenopathy. Nodes can also be a site for cancers, the most frequent of which is lymphoma. Lymph nodes are found everywhere in the body and are designated based on the anatomical region in which they are found; the principal types of nodes are cervical, inguinal, abdominal, and thoracic.

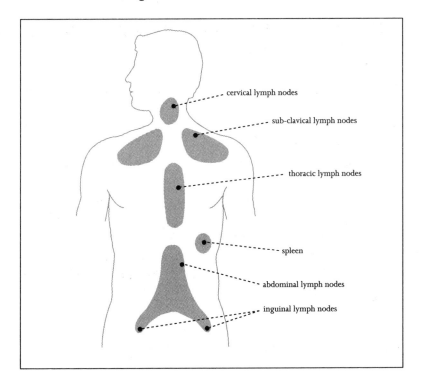

cervical lymph nodes

sub-clavical lymph nodes

thoracic lymph nodes

spleen

abdominal lymph nodes

inguinal lymph nodes

Lymphatic Ducts

Lymphatic ducts are the small vessels that link nodes together. When an infection is present, the white cells travel through these ducts to reach the nodes, where they multiply to better fight the infection. When a cancer is present, this circuit often serves as a way for the malignant tumor to spread. Cancerous cells can detach from the tumor and use the lymphatic ducts to invade regional nodes, thus forming node metastases.

Spleen

The spleen resembles a small blood-filled bag and is approximately the same size as a tomato. It is located on the left side of the abdomen and, like a tomato, is very fragile.

Its main role is eliminating "old red blood cells," those that have carried oxygen for more than 120 days and are beginning to age. The spleen recognizes them and picks them out of the blood supply.

It also plays an important part in the fight against infections by eliminating bacteria and particulate antigens from the bloodstream. Several diseases can cause the spleen to increase in volume (splenomegaly); the most common are viral infections, liver diseases, inflammatory diseases, and malignant diseases such as leukemia and lymphoma. Under such circumstances, the spleen can swell to the size of a football; when it does, it is extremely vulnerable to the slightest trauma.

The Cardiorespiratory System

The cardiorespiratory system is composed mainly of the heart, the lungs, and the large blood vessels.

The heart is an organ whose role is to ensure good blood circulation to all parts of our bodies. It is divided into two parts: the right heart and the left heart.

The right heart receives nonoxygenated blood from our muscles and our organs; this blood travels through the venous system and ends up in the superior and inferior vena cava. The right heart pumps this blood to the lungs.

The lungs ensure that gases are exchanged and that the blood is reoxygenated, turning bright red in the process.

The left heart pumps the oxygenated blood to all organs in our body. The heart beats more than 100,000 times in one day; it adjusts its rhythm and the strength of its contractions constantly, reflecting changes in the demand for oxygen.

Some hematological conditions can increase cardiac rhythm, such as a patient suffering from anemia or an infection.

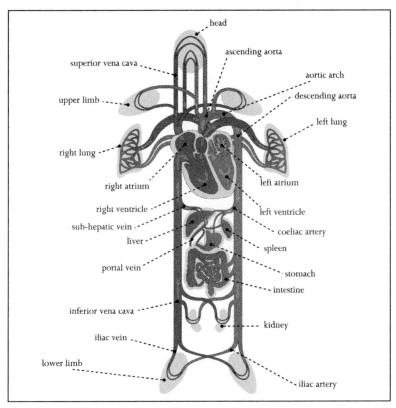

The cardiorespiratory system

The Central Nervous System

The central nervous system is a series of organs composed of nervous tissues, all of them closely linked to each other. It includes the brain, the cerebellum, the brain stem, and the spinal cord.

The brain, the cerebellum, and the brain stem group together millions of cells called neurons. These cells cannot multiply and they communicate with one another through a system of branching parts whose total length can go to beyond one meter.

The spinal cord is formed by this system of branching parts, which travels through the center of vertebra in a canal known as the vertebral canal. The spinal cord is divided into several sections, which are known as nerves. A break in the spinal cord results in irreversible paralysis. The central nervous system is enveloped in cerebrospinal fluid,

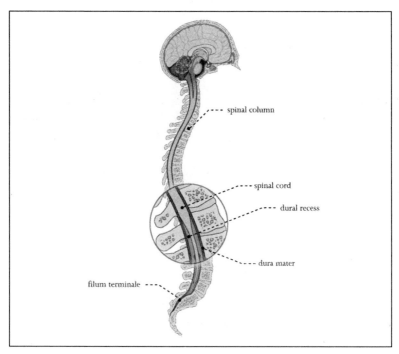

spinal column

spinal cord

dural recess

dura mater

filum terminale

The central nervous system

which circulates constantly while protecting and nourishing it. When a physician proceeds with a lumbar puncture, he removes several milliliters of cerebrospinal fluid.

Several malignant blood diseases tend to spread to the central nervous system, in particular, childhood leukemia. Analysis of the cerebrospinal fluid makes it possible to detect the presence of leukemic cells and, consequently, to modify treatment programs; if cancerous cells are present or to prevent certain types of leukemia, the central nervous system will be treated with radiation, and chemotherapy drugs will be injected directly into the cerebrospinal fluid (intrathecal injection).

The Digestive System

The digestive system includes the digestive tract and several organs, each of which has a specific part to play in food digestion.

The Digestive Tract

The digestive tract extends from the mouth to the anus and its main role is to digest and absorb food. In this complex process, each part of the digestive tract has a very specific function.

The inside of the digestive tract is lined with a thin layer of cells, called intestinal mucous membrane. These cells characteristically multiply very quickly; therefore, they are very sensitive to cancer-fighting treatments.

In the mouth, food is chewed and mixed with saliva from the salivary glands. The food is then swallowed, passing through the esophagus on its way to the stomach. Chemotherapy and radiation therapy can affect the salivary glands and the taste buds (small glands located on the tongue and used to taste food); patients will have difficulty tasting foods and will have dry mouths. A mucositis (red blotches and a burning sensation in the mouth) and an esophagitis (irritation of the esophagus caused by burning when food is swallowed) can sometimes occur.

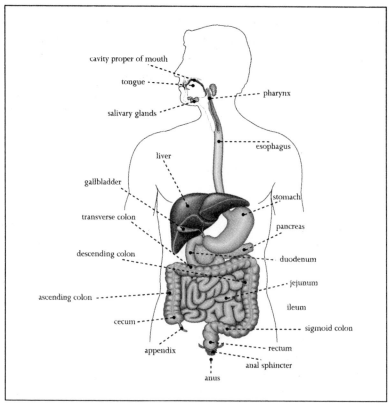

The digestive system

The stomach is a reservoir where food is stored for a few hours. The food is mixed with a very acidic liquid that breaks it down and prepares it for absorption. The stomach is sensitive to certain medications (aspirin, cortisone) and can react to stress by increasing its acid level; this reaction can degenerate into gastritis (irritation of the stomach, causing heartburn, which can be relieved temporarily by drinking milk or water) and sometimes even ulcers (deep erosion of the stomach wall). If not treated quickly, gastritis and ulcers can lead to stomach hemorrhages. In response to certain medications, to stress, and to inflammation, the stomach's movements may be upset and the person will experience nausea and, on occasion, vomiting.

The duodenum, the small intestine, and the large intestine form a tube approximately 21 feet (seven meters) long. Solid food is absorbed in the small intestine, and liquids are absorbed in the large intestine.

During anticancer treatment, the mucous membrane in this region commonly stops its absorption activities; as a result, the patient may experience severe diarrhea. The physician can sometimes counter this lack of food absorption by feeding the patient intravenously.

All of the side effects that chemotherapy can have on the digestive tract are reversible as soon as the treatment program ends.

The Pancreas
This organ has two different functions. The first is to take part in the digestive process by producing pancreatic juices, which are emptied into the duodenum. These juices contain enzymes essential to the digestion of meats, sugars, and fats. Its second function consists of secreting hormones, the most well known of which is insulin (which maintains proper glucose levels in the blood; a decrease in the secretion of insulin leads to diabetes).

The pancreas can be damaged by certain substances, such as alcohol or medications, or by stones that block its opening and cause congestion and inflammation of the pancreas (pancreatitis). Cases of pancreatitis are rare during anticancer treatment programs.

The Liver
The liver is the organ with the highest number of functions to provide. First, it participates in the digestion of food by secreting bile. Essential for the digestion of fats, bile is stored in the gallbladder before emptying into the duodenum. The liver also manufactures a number of proteins, the most important of which are albumin and blood coagulation proteins, vital to the formation of blood clots. In addition, it helps to eliminate organic wastes and medications from the body; its role in anticancer treatment programs is extremely important.

The liver is sensitive to several medications, to toxic substances, and even to some viruses. An obstruction in the bile ducts, often caused by gallbladder stones and, more rarely, by tumors (lymphoma or cancer of the pancreas), creates congestion of the liver. When the liver is inflamed by one of the previously mentioned causes, the condition is known as hepatitis.

During chemotherapy, the liver is kept under close watch since medication-related hepatitis is frequent; blood tests are taken regularly, and at the first sign of damage, treatment is modified or stopped.

The liver can be affected by certain malignant blood diseases, such as various forms of leukemia and lymphoma, and at times, in instances of bone marrow transplants, by the graft versus host reaction (see "The GVH Reaction" in Chapter 5); the physician proceeds with a biopsy to confirm or invalidate the diagnosis.

The Urinary System

The urinary system mainly includes the kidneys, the urethra, and the bladder. The kidneys play a key role in the elimination of medications and biological wastes produced from our various organs.

The Kidneys

Among other functions, the kidneys balance arterial pressure and adjust the quantity of liquid and the level of minerals (sodium, potassium, calcium, chlorides, etc.) present in our bodies and essential for the proper functioning of our organs. They are also involved in the elimination of organic wastes (urea) and medications, which they concentrate and eliminate in the urine.

The kidneys are rarely affected by malignant blood diseases, but they are very sensitive to certain anticancer or antirejection medications, such as cyclosporin. During anticancer treatment programs the kidneys are monitored closely (for example, through regular blood tests and urine analyses).

If a medication changes kidney functions, its dosage is immediately decreased; at times, the physician may stop administering the medication completely, replacing it with an alternative that is less toxic for the kidneys.

The Bladder

Urine that is synthesized in the kidneys travels through the urethra to the bladder. The latter acts as a reservoir; when its maximum storage capacity is reached, sensors located along its wall send a message to the central nervous system, which warns us that urination is imminent.

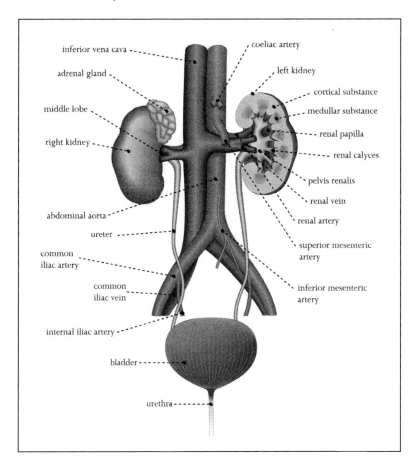

inferior vena cava
coeliac artery
adrenal gland
left kidney
middle lobe
cortical substance
medullar substance
renal papilla
right kidney
renal calyces
pelvis renalis
renal vein
abdominal aorta
renal artery
ureter
superior mesenteric artery
common iliac artery
common iliac vein
inferior mesenteric artery
internal iliac artery
bladder
urethra

The urinary system

As we have seen, urine can contain several medication residues; occasionally, some of these can cause an irritation of the bladder (medication-related cystitis). Sometimes, bacteria and viruses infect the bladder (infectious cystitis) and can even travel backward through the urethra to infect the kidneys (pyelonephritis). Infectious cystitis and pyelonephritis can be treated quickly with antibiotics.

The Blood Test

The blood test is a simple test that makes it possible to evaluate the functioning of most organs. In hematology, the blood test is used to evaluate the condition, type, and number of blood cells; this evaluation constitutes a detailed cellular profile.

Understanding a Detailed Cellular Profile

The detailed cellular profile is the calculation and analysis of the different cells present in approximately two cubic centimeters of blood.

The results of the profile are presented in a chart (see the next page) that provides a range of information on the quantity, type, shape, and even contents of cells. Some of this information is pertinent only to medical experts and specialists, but as you can see, some of it is very general and will help you to understand the composition of blood.

The profile involves two steps. In the first step, which is mechanical, a machine counts the various cells and calculates the hemoglobin level (Part A of the profile); the machine then separates the various types of white cells and gives the result in percentages (Part B of the profile, referred to as differential).

Report on the Cellular Profile

Part A

Number of white blood cells (polynuclears, neutrophils, lymphocytes, and all other white blood cells)

Number of red blood cells

Hemoglobin

Number of platelets

Part B

Differential:

- Neutrophil
- Lymphocyte

These blood cells are rare and their presence is linked to several disorders, including infections and blood diseases.

Note that the number of white blood cells must be multiplied by a factor of 1,000 to obtain the number of blood cells per cubic millimeter.

Results of the patient's test | ***Normal values*** | ***Description of certain cells under microscope*** | ***Part C***

FSC	CODES	NORMAL
•	White $\times 10^9$/L	4.5 -10.0
•	Red $\times 10^{12}$/L	W 4.0 - 5.4 M 4.6 - 6.1
•	HB g/L	W 120 - 160 M 140 - 180
•	HT	W .37 - .47 M .42 - .50
•	VGM fl	80 - 99.9
•	HGM Pg	27 - 32
•	CHGM g/L	330 - 360
•	RDW	13.0 ± 1.5
•	Platelets $\times 10^9$/L	130 - 450
•	VPM	8.9 ± 1.5
•	Lympho. %	20 - 40
•	Mono. %	5 - 10
•	Gran. %	50 - 70
•	Lympho. $\times 10^9$	.8 - 4.0
•	Mono. $\times 10^9$	.2 - 1.0
•	Gran. x 10₉	2.3 - 7.6

Anisocytosis	
Poikilocytosis	
Hypochromia	
Microcytosis	
Macrocytosis	
Polychrom.	
Target cells	
Ovalocytes	
Elliptocytes	
C. Burr	
Acanthocytes	
Schistocytes	
Dacryocytes	
Gr. creneles	
Rolls	
Howell-Jolly	
Gran. Baso.	
Stomatocytes	
Spherocytes	
Red masses	
Anisochromia	

DIFFERENTIAL	%	NORMAL	9 9 9 9 9 9 9	
Neutrophil		55 - 65	Toxic gran.	
Lymphocyte		25 - 35	Hyper segmented	
Monocyte		3 - 7	Bilobed	
Eosinophilic		1 - 5	Dahle	
Basophile		0 - 1	Auer	
Stab		1 - 5		
Metamyelocyte		0	Sedimentation	
Myelocyte		0	Norm	
Promyelocyte		0	M 0 - 20	
Blast		0	W 0 - 10	
Atypical lymphocyte		0	Reticulocytes	
Plasmocyte		0	N: 0.5 - 2.5	
Smudge		0	No.	

The second step is carried out by a hematologist, who looks directly at cells using a microscope. He or she verifies the accuracy of the machine's analysis and notes certain additional observations in Part C of the profile.

The description of the cells, in Parts B and C, is specific to certain diseases; it helps the physician confirm the diagnosis, but is much too specialized to delve into in detail here. We will examine only the most pertinent results to arrive at an overall understanding of the cellular profile. Readers who are particularly curious can ask their physicians any additional questions they may have.

Factors that lead to an increase in the number of white cells	• Infections • Inflammatory diseases • Major traumas (severe burns, traffic accidents, etc.) • Certain medications (cortisone) • Blood diseases (various forms of leukemia)
Factors that lead to a decrease in the number of white cells	• Certain severe infections early in their development • Advanced states of malnutrition • Liver diseases • Anticancer medications and treatments • Malignant blood diseases (forms of leukemia, aplasia, lymphoma)
Factors that lead to an increase in the hemoglobin level	• Excessive smoking • Blood diseases (Vaquez disease) • Decrease in the total quantity of plasma (dehydration)
Factors that lead to anemia (decrease in the hemoglobin level)	• Hemorrhages • Hemolysis (premature destruction of red cells) • Increase in the plasma level (pregnancy) • Iron, vitamin B_{12}, or folic acid deficiency • Inflammatory diseases • Renal insufficiency • Thyroid gland disease • Anticancer medications and treatments • Blood diseases (forms of leukemia, aplasia, lymphoma) • Presence of a cancer unrelated to the blood

Factors that lead to an increase in the number of platelets	• Certain infections • Severe traumas (burns, traffic accidents, etc.) • Certain types of leukemia
Factors that lead to a decrease in the number of platelets	• Certain severe infections • Inflammatory diseases • Liver disease • Anticancer medications and treatments • Malignant blood disease and cancers of other origins
Factors that lead to an increase in the number of neutrophils	• Infections of bacterial origin • Inflammatory diseases • Myelogenous-type leukemia
Factors that lead to an increase in the number of lymphocytes	• Infections of viral origin • Lymphoid-type leukemia • Lymphomas and rejection reactions
Factors that lead to a decrease in the number of neutrophils and lymphocytes	• Same as those leading to a decrease in the number of white cells

Bone Marrow Puncture and the Bone Biopsy

Bone marrow in the sternum and the hip bone contains the highest number of stem cells. Hematologists describe the marrow in these bones as "rich."

The physician extracts marrow through a medullar puncture in the pelvis and the sternum, regions that are easily accessible and whose bones provide a high number of stem cells. The stem cells collected in the process are then submitted to a range of analyses conducted in a hematology laboratory.

The bone biopsy is an examination practiced simultaneously and allows the laboratory to do a complementary study of the marrow. The patient lies face-down on a bed or examination table. The procedure lasts only a few minutes and involves very little pain. The patient can get up and leave immediately after the procedure is completed.

It is important not to confuse bone marrow with the spinal cord; the spinal cord is a continuation of the brain, composed of nervous tissue that runs through the center of the spinal column and is divided between vertebra, forming nerves. A lesion of the spinal cord results in paralysis of the entire part of the body located below the lesion.

Complications that may occur during bone marrow puncture or a bone biopsy are benign; on rare occasions, there may be some bruising or small local skin infections.

Steps in the Procedure

Step 1: The area is disinfected with iodine and local anesthesia is administered.

The iodine eliminates bacteria on the skin and prevents infection. Local anesthesia is administered by injecting a few cubic centimeters of liquid (xylocaine) under the skin and on the bone. As a result of the anesthesia, inserting the needle and trocar used during the puncture and the biopsy is a painless process.

Step 2: The needle is inserted into the bone, reaching the bone marrow (one cubic centimeter of bone marrow is aspirated, and part of it is examined under a microscope).

Step 3: The trocar is inserted and a small cylinder (one or two centimeters) is filled with marrow.

Lumbar Puncture

A lumbar puncture, also called rachicentesis, is an operation that consists of collecting the liquid surrounding the spinal cord (cerebrospinal fluid) to analyze its contents and arrive at a diagnosis. The procedure is simple, involves very little pain, and takes only a few minutes. It can be done while the patient is seated or lying down, but it is important for the patient to arch his or her back, providing a maximum opening between vertebrae, where the puncture is made.

After applying a local anesthetic to the skin, the physician introduces a fine needle between two vertebrae to reach the cerebrospinal fluid, removing a few cubic centimeters of the liquid.

In the case of a cancer investigation, the presence of cancerous cells in the liquid indicates that the disease has spread to the central nervous system. In the case of an investigation surrounding an infection, the presence of numerous white cells and bacteria indicates an infection of the vertebral canal (meningitis).

A lumbar puncture also makes it possible to introduce certain medications (chemotherapy drugs, antibiotics) to fight a disease more effectively.

After a lumbar puncture, it is important that the patient remain lying on his or her back for a few hours. This prevents liquid from escaping through the puncture site, which would result in a headache.

X-ray Examinations

In the case of blood diseases, physicians use standard X-rays, ultrasonography, and computerized tomography (scanners), especially in the investigation of lymphomas and infections. Magnetic resonance imaging is similar to computerized tomography; this method is particularly efficient to detect lesions of the nervous system.

Nuclear Medicine

Nuclear medicine is used to examine how organs function and the various inflammatory reactions that accompany certain diseases.

It is possible to identify the site and extent of an infection or a tumor, to diagnose a pulmonary embolism, or to see how the kidneys, heart, liver, and brain are functioning using coloring agents that emit low levels of radiation (harmless to the body) and that are specifically designed to penetrate these particular organs.

Step 1: Nuclear medicine examinations are painless. A radioactive coloring agent designed to penetrate a particular site is injected into a vein.

Step 2: The patient must wait patiently; sometimes it takes several hours before the coloring agent penetrates the target site completely.

Step 3: The patient lies down or stands, depending on the target site, while a sensor attached to the site analyzes the weak emissions of the coloring agent.

Surgery and Diagnosis

An accurate diagnosis is crucial in the choice of the appropriate treatment program. Surgery is vital in the diagnosis of several diseases, in particular those that affect the lymph nodes.

Examining a swollen lymph node (lymphadenopathy) requires taking a sample and studying it under a microscope. When the surgeon performs a lymph node biopsy, the patient is taken to an operating room and, depending on the location of the affected node, samples are taken under local or general anesthesia. Usually, the patient tolerates the surgery very well.

Sometimes, the exploration can require a laparotomy. The laparotomy is an abdominal operation during which the surgeon explores various organs visually and manually; if some of the organs seem abnormal, biopsies are done at the same time. A surgical procedure of the same type, the thoracotomy, is sometimes used to explore the thorax. However, in the case of diseases that affect the lymph nodes, very little surgery is used for curative purposes, since they tend to spread to several organs at once, which makes surgery impossible.

Malignant Blood Diseases   4

The blood diseases we will discuss in this chapter all involve a high risk of death if they are not treated quickly and appropriately; for this reason, they are known as *malignant* diseases. In contrast, diseases referred to as *benign* are a less severe threat to a patient.

For example, if through palpation a physician discovers a small lump in a woman's breast, it will be described as a tumor. But the medical term *tumor* is simply used to designate a lump. Only after a biopsy and a reading of the pathologist's report can the physician specify whether the tumor is benign (noncancerous, meaning this is a case of a fibrocytic disease of the breast, or a lipoma) or malignant (cancer of the breast).

First, we will look at what cancer is and we will examine the mechanisms that can cause it; then we will study malignant blood diseases.

Cancer

What Is Cancer?

Cancer is an uninterrupted multiplication of cells that eventually fills all of the space around them.

All of the body's organs can generate "malignant" cells; however, some organs have a greater propensity to develop cancers. Thus, cancers of the skin, lungs, breast, intestines, and prostate are the most common; in the case of blood cancer, we speak of leukemia, lymphoma, myeloblastic syndromes, and myeloma.

At times, cancerous cells group together in bunches and form a malignant tumor that may compress adjacent organs. For example, some tumors of the abdomen can compress large blood vessels and jeopardize circulation, which causes an accumulation of fluid in the legs (edema) and in the abdomen (ascites).

Metastases

Cancer cells can detach themselves from the main tumor and attach themselves to other areas, such as the liver or the lungs; in these cases, they form hepatic (liver) or pulmonary metastases. If several organs are affected at the same time, we refer to generalized metastases; some people use the term generalized cancer.

Malignant cells multiply nonstop, consume a great deal of energy, and often exhaust patients' reserves, at which point they begin to lose weight and to weaken for no apparent reason.

The symptoms patients present are linked to the type, extent, and location of the cancer.

Causes of Cancer

The exact causes of cancer remain unknown. We know that there are many factors that increase the risk of cancer (see "The Factors Linked to Cancer," pages 89–92), such as smoking, certain chemical products, and radiation. But the cause-and-effect link between these factors and the formation of a cancer is not well understood.

Recent discoveries in molecular biology lead us to believe that the abnormality in cells that have become cancerous occurs in the genes located inside the nucleus of the cells.

The Theory of Molecular Biology: Genetic Instability

Inside the nucleus, and more specifically on the DNA chain (the chain that contains the genetic code), researchers recently discovered certain genes that were linked to the transformation of normal cells into cancerous cells. The most crucial change associated with cancer is genetic instability, which leads to dysregulation of gene function and cell growth. Some genes (called oncogenes) that enhance cell proliferation become more active, while other genes (called tumor suppressor genes) are turned off.

This discovery is extremely important, because we have long known that the DNA chain coordinates all of the cell's work, including the cell's own multiplication. The idea that a faulty gene could be the underlying cause in the development of a cancer had been under consideration for a long time, but the hypothesis had never been proven until this discovery was made.

To date, researchers have identified a high number of oncogenes, including several that are linked with malignant blood diseases. Following is a list of the main oncogenes.

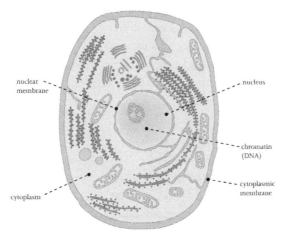

nuclear membrane

nucleus

chromatin (DNA)

cytoplasmic membrane

cytoplasm

The cell, the nucleus and the genes

87

Oncogenes	*Associated Cancer*
c-myc	Lines produced by leukemia and pulmonary carcinoma in humans
"	Lymphoma in chickens
N-myc	Neuroblastoma and retinoblastoma in humans
L-myc	Small-cell pulmonary cancer in humans
c-abl	Line produced by chronic myelogenous leukemia in humans
c-myb	Lines produced by acute myelogenous leukemia and carcinoma of the colon
c-erbB	Line produced by epidermoid carcinoma in humans
c-K-ras	Line produced by carcinoma of the colon in humans
"	Line produced by adrenocortical carcinoma in mice

Note that certain oncogenes are present in different types of cancer found in humans. They can even be present in various types of cancer found in animals. Therefore, oncogenes are a key factor in the development of cancer.

The initial studies showing that the transformation of a gene can lead to cancer were made using viruses that produced cancers in animals. Known as retroviruses, they are able to penetrate a cell and incorporate their own genes into the cell's DNA. While these viral genes are minuscule, their introduction at a particular location on the DNA can modify the code of the gene in which they have been incorporated; furthermore, they can modify the code of an adjacent gene.

Viruses are not the only agents capable of modifying genes; several factors (see "The Factors Linked to Cancer" on the next page) can cause breaks and rearrangements in genes (mutations). The mutation of a gene can modify the DNA code and transmit an erroneous command to the cell, such as the command to divide nonstop.

Therefore, the oncogene is a gene that was normal, but that has been modified (by a retrovirus or mutation) and now transmits an erroneous message to the cell. This message constitutes a command: to multiply nonstop. Consequently, the oncogene leads to the malignant transformation of this particular cell.

The Factors Linked to Cancer

Every day, we come into contact with more than 6,000 potentially carcinogenic products. These substances vary: synthetic coloring used in foods or cosmetic products; food preservatives; artificial sweeteners; chemical fertilizers; herbicides; insecticides; air pollutants; water pollutants; fumes from gas, paints, solvents; various products such as alcohol and tobacco, and other substances too numerous to mention— the list could easily fill this entire book!

How have these products infiltrated our daily lives over the years?

The best way to understand the complexity of this topic is to look at the history of synthetic coloring agents, as told by Fernand Séguin in La Bombe et l'Orchidée (The Bomb and the Orchid):

> Group behavior has the peculiarity of obliterating the type of reasoning that individuals usually present when they act calmly. In other words, a crowd never acts cool-headedly.
>
> When it comes to collective phobias, regarding cancer or contagious diseases such as AIDS, we can see how excessive public opinion is, especially when it is fuelled by the media.
>
> In 1960, a phobia began to take shape around the subject of synthetic coloring agents used in food products and cosmetics as diverse as maraschino cherries, lollipops, children's cereals and even lipstick.
>
> The focus was on finding some form of protection against cancer, on exorcising the collective fear.
>
> To appease cancer phobics, 200 of these coloring agents were banned by the U.S. Food and Drug Administration, based on proof that they were carcinogenic when administered in high doses to laboratory animals.

The ban was legislated in the form of a now famous amendment, the Delaney Amendment, which stipulated that "The Secretary [of the Food and Drug Administration] shall not approve for use in food any chemical additive found to induce cancer in man or, after tests, found to induce cancer in animals." The assumption was that the only safe dose is zero.

The measure was excessive but it contributed to reassuring public opinion; this is all that mattered to public officials, accustomed to intervening only under the pressure of the circumstances.

Over the course of subsequent years and at the insistence of manufacturers, the list of 200 banished coloring agents was cut down to 63, then to 6, all of which are shades of red, though no one fears them any longer.

How did these coloring agents come to be considered inoffensive? Simply because public administrators, docile in the face of arguments presented by manufacturers, introduced the notion of "acceptable risk." There was no claim that synthetic coloring agents had lost their toxicity; the claim was that the risk of contracting some form of cancer while eating red-colored candy or using red lipstick was so low, it was best forgotten. For its part, the Delaney Amendment still exists as is, but each time a faction calls for its application, another demands more experimental proof of harmful effects.

The first lesson to be learned from this story is that collective phobias (and these phobias spread in a mysterious way) can result in laws whose rigorousness has nothing in common with the complexity of reality. Once the phobia fades, we can change course without creating any major waves.

The second reflection is that collective phobias are as big a threat as the dangers that serve as their focus.

In our day-to-day environment, both individual and collective, we come into contact with thousands of substances that are recognized as potentially carcinogenic. It would be illusion and folly to want to eliminate them all—others would replace them.

> Limiting ourselves to the food industry, we should ask ourselves
> what led us to ask for yellow butter, pink ham, bread as white as
> chalk. Real butter isn't yellow, ham isn't pink and real bread is
> slightly gray.
> It may be that manufacturers, in collusion with advertising
> experts, are selling us just about anything under false appearances. It
> may be that having lost the memory of the color and taste of things,
> we have become involuntary accomplices in their degradation.

In this era of communication, in which we watch wars, famines, and cataclysms live on television, unbeknown to ourselves we are becoming increasingly insensitive to the many things we see. We remain insensitive until we personally face an ordeal or a catastrophe, at which point our values and our ability for reflection and analysis come to the fore once again.

With regard to environmental issues, for example, our perception of water and air pollution has become concrete, instantaneous, and linked to very specific images. For a very significant portion of the population, water pollution is a tanker spilling its cargo on a faraway shore, coating ducks and seals in thick, black oil. Live television reports quantify the disaster in terms of thousands of barrels or hundreds of ducks and, in a few days, nothing else is heard until the next mega-incident. No wonder we pay no attention to reports of toxic products accidentally spilled into a river that runs through our own community or to a warning that a local beach is off limits to swimmers because the water is contaminated with coliform bacteria.

Our idea of air pollution is the odor from automobile and bus exhaust systems, the carbon dioxide level, and the parts per million recorded at rush hour. But there are also the quantities of benzene, PCBs, heavy metals, insecticides, pesticides, and chemical industrial derivatives found in the water we drink and the air we breathe.

Unless there is an ecological disaster of some sort, these items are rarely mentioned in weather bulletins, since these odorless and colorless substances are present at levels well under the tolerated norms and, therefore, constitute an acceptable risk for our health. We live in a world of "acceptable risks"; however, if misfortune strikes and we are stricken with cancer, for example, we no longer consider statistics and risks as acceptable. Suddenly, we are aware of all the toxic substances that surround us in microquantities.

The cumulative effects these substances have on our bodies are unknown. In medical terms, we designate these cumulative effects using the term *synergism*: two products used separately have a known and quantified effect on the body, but when they are used simultaneously, their effect is five times greater. As an example, take smoking and asbestos. It is well known that these two factors increase the risk of lung cancer. But when asbestos workers smoke, their risk of contracting cancer is much higher than the simple calculation of the combined risk of the two factors.

Taken separately, toxic products X and Y, found in small quantities in the environment, present a risk deemed to be acceptable for the population's health. But if X and Y are found together at a given time in the water we drink or the air we breathe, their synergetic effect can be excessively toxic for our bodies.

The synergetic effect of certain products may be at the root of a number of diseases; within our cells, they may even cause mutations that may lead to cancer.

Several factors are recognized for their strong link to certain types of cancer found in humans. The table on the next page shows the main cancer-causing agents, many of which are found in our day-to-day lives.

Nutrition and Cancer

Excessive consumption of alcohol is linked to cancer of the larynx, pharynx, esophagus, stomach, and liver. Certain types of alcohol are more harmful than others; for example, the Japanese drink a lot of hot rice wine (sake), which leads to an increase in cancer of the esophagus.

The Factors Linked to Cancer in Humans

Agents	Type of exposure	Cancer sites
Nutrition and smoking		
Alcohol	Excessive consumption	pharynx, larynx, esophagus, stomach, liver
Foods rich in fat	Excessive meat consumption	colon
Tobacco	Smoking, especially cigarettes	lung, pharynx, larynx, esophagus, pancreas, bladder, kidney
Infections		
Viruses	Epstein-Barr virus	Burkitt's lymphoma
	HTLV-1 virus	(T)lymphocytic leukemia
	Hepatitis B virus	liver
	HIV virus (AIDS)	Kaposi's sarcoma lymphoma
	Papillomavirus and Type II herpes	cervix
Parasites	Schistosomiasis	bladder
Drugs		
Chemotherapy (alkylant agents)	medication	leukemia
Immunosuppressives	antirejection medication	lymphoma, skin sarcoma
Anabolic steroids	to increase muscle mass (drugs used by athletes)	liver
Industrial and mining products		
Benzene	oil, paint, dye	leukemia
Arsenic	mining products, pesticides, contaminated water	lung, skin, liver
Asbestos	mining and processing products (insulating products)	liver, pleura, peritoneum, intestine
Hydrocarbons	coal, petroleum products	lung, skin
Vinyls and aromatic amines	chemical industry	bladder
Radiation		
Ultraviolet	exposure to the sun	skin
Ionizing	atomic bomb, accidental leaks from nuclear power stations or medical use	all types of cancer

Consumed in excessive quantities, alcohol irritates the digestive system's mucous membrane. Cells that react to an irritation tend to multiply rapidly, to change their usual behavior patterns, and to become precancerous (metaplasia). If the excessive alcohol consumption persists, some of the cells will become malignant and will form a tumor.

The consumption of fats and meat in large quantities, coupled with a diet low in fiber, increases the risk of intestinal cancer. North Americans, for example, are the world's biggest meat consumers, and they also have the highest rate of colon cancer. Toxins generated by the digestion of fats and meat are an irritant for the intestine and cause metaplasia of the mucous membrane. A diet rich in fiber has the opposite effect because it facilitates the evacuation of these toxins and, thus, decreases the risk of intestinal cancer.

Studies have shown that obese women are more susceptible to cancers of the uterus and breast; the cause is attributed to consumption of foods rich in fat and the increase in estrogen that results from an increase in weight.

The lack of certain types of food in our diet has the effect of increasing the risk of certain cancers (see table on next page). Thus, a diet poor in vitamin A (carrots) and selenium is linked to high levels of lung cancer, a deficiency in vitamin C (fruit and vegetables) increases the risk of stomach cancer, and eating raw vegetables decreases the risk of intestinal cancer.

Therefore, it is possible to reduce the risk of cancer through a healthy diet. We suggest a balanced diet that is rich in fiber, fruit, and vegetables. Limit the amount of food you cook over charcoal and limit consumption of fried foods. And, of course, restrict your consumption of meat and alcohol.

Smoking

The risk of cancers of the larynx, pharynx, lungs, esophagus, bladder, kidneys, and pancreas is increased among smokers and individuals

Food and Cancer

Foods	Effects on cancer
Coffee	No study has shown a specific link with cancer, but a few inconclusive studies indicate a possible increase in cancer of the bladder and pancreas; however, the cause-and-effect link has not been proven.
Animal fats	Increase in the risk of intestinal cancer: animal fats increase the secretion of bile acids in the intestine and these acids are then transformed by bacteria; certain carcinogenic substances (nitrosamines) are released during the transformation process.
Fiber	Decreases the risk of intestinal cancer: fiber increases the size of the food ball and carries it, so intestinal evacuation is quicker, which decreases the concentration of carcinogenic toxins released by bacteria in the intestine.
Artificial food colorings	Linked to cancers in laboratory animals when they are ingested in very high doses.
Artificial sweeteners (saccharines, cyclamates)	Linked to cancers of the bladder in laboratory animals; the risk for humans is considered very low.
Iodine	Iodine, found in raw vegetables (broccoli, brussels sprouts, cauliflower), decreases the risk of intestinal cancer and inhibits carcinogens secreted by intestinal bacteria.
Vitamin A	This vitamin, found in carrots, decreases the risk of lung cancer, but the action mechanism is unknown.
Vitamin C	This vitamin decreases the risk of stomach cancer by inhibiting the formation of nitrosamines (carcinogenic substances). It is found in fruit (oranges, grapefruit, lemons) and vegetables.
Cooking methods	While not proven, researchers believe that cooking food over charcoal or at high temperatures could produce carcinogens and increase the risk of certain types of cancer.

exposed to secondhand smoke over a number of years. It is estimated that smoking causes 30 percent of all cancers, among men and women alike. Smokers are twenty times more likely to contract lung cancer than are nonsmokers.

Smoking increases cancer rates in two ways: through local irritation and through toxins. Smoke causes an inflammation (irritation) of the respiratory system's walls (throat, vocal cords, trachea, bronchi). After a few years of exposure to smoke, these walls are inevitably affected by metaplasia. If the exposure to smoke does not stop, cancerous transformation can occur. In addition, as cigarettes burn they release several types of toxins (tar, products resulting from burning paper, etc.) that are inhaled into the lungs and that penetrate the body. In the long run, these toxins can cause cancer in certain internal organs such as the bladder, the kidneys, and the pancreas.

Infections

There is a proven link between certain viral infectious agents and cancer. The Epstein-Barr virus causes mononucleosis among Western populations and is linked to Burkitt's lymphoma in Africa's black populations. The HTLV-1 virus (human T lymphotrophic virus) is linked to (T)lymphocytic leukemia in Japan and the Caribbean. The hepatitis B virus is linked to liver cancer among Asians and Africans. The HIV virus (human immunodeficiency virus) causes AIDS and is linked to Kaposi's sarcoma and to non-Hodgkin lymphoma. Papillomavirus and Type II herpes simplex are two sexually transmitted viruses that, if not treated, increase the risk of cancer of the cervix over the long term.

The mechanisms of cancerous transformation linked to these viruses are not well known. We believe that the viruses in question can incorporate themselves into the genes of cells and create mutations or oncogenes that result in the malignance of the cells. They also may act by weakening our immune system, which then loses its capacity to recognize and destroy malignant cells.

Schistosomiasis is a common disease in the Middle East and North Africa. A parasite infects the bladder and, over the long term, results in cancer of the bladder.

Ionizing Radiation

Ionizing radiation (X-rays, electrons, and gamma rays) consists of invisible rays that travel at extremely high speeds; these rays are produced by the disintegration of certain radioactive minerals, the most well known being uranium and radium. Ionizing radiation is divided into two categories: low-energy radiation and high-energy radiation.

Whether low-energy or high-energy, ionizing radiation breaks down the long DNA chain of cells (see "The Cell" in Chapter 2) and, consequently, creates potential mutations. The latter are linked to the cancerous transformation; our cells are capable of absorbing a certain number of mutations without any damage to our health, but if the number of mutations reaches a critical level, the risk of cancer is higher. Furthermore, if the breaks in the DNA chain are countless, the cell will die. This phenomenon is the basis of radiotherapy treatment (see Chapter 5).

Low-energy Radiation
This type of radiation is used in diagnostic radiology and nuclear medicine. The radiation doses emitted by X-rays during routine medical examinations are very low, and therefore the risk of creating mutations is infinitesimal, virtually nonexistent.

Even though the risk involved in a diagnostic X-ray is minimal, the physician will always take the time to weigh the risk against the benefits the examination will bring to the patient. No examination, even if it presents virtually no risk, has a place in a diagnostic process if it does not provide additional information to the physician.

High-energy Radiation
This type of radiation is used in radiotherapy. It is also produced by the nuclear fission used in nuclear power plants, in turbines used in submarines or boats, and in the atomic bomb.

When high-energy radiation is controlled and concentrated on only one area of the body, as in the case of radiotherapy treatment directed on a cancerous tumor, the energy of this radiation causes countless breaks in the DNA chain, which destroys the malignant cells in the irradiated area. High-energy radiation concentrated on a precise region has a beneficial effect in the treatment of cancer. However, if it is not controlled, radiation can be extremely dangerous for our health.

The same holds true for radiation from nuclear accidents (nuclear power stations, the atomic bomb, nuclear waste, the irradiation of workers and miners who work with radioactive minerals), since this type of radiation usually has enough energy to penetrate the body and create mutations inside cells. These mutations can lead to cancers, even several years after the irradiation occurs, and almost all types of cancer increase under such circumstances.

Examples of irradiation experienced by large populations include that caused by the atomic bombs dropped on Hiroshima and Nagasaki during World War II and, more recently, accidents at nuclear power stations at Three Mile Island in 1979 and Chernobyl in 1986. These accidents caused a strong increase in cancers of the thyroid and breast as well as leukemia among people living up to several dozens of miles from the accident site—in other words, people who had received only small doses of radiation.

People located very close to the disaster sites suffered skin burns identical to sunburn; for several, the radiation was so strong that bone marrow (which is very sensitive to radiation) was destroyed due to the countless breaks in the DNA chain of stem cells. These people died of aplasia in the days following the irradiation.

It is estimated that at the time of the disaster at Chernobyl (although not all information is available), more than six hundred of the eight hundred workers assigned to the power station died of aplasia in the weeks following the accident. In the area immediately surrounding Chernobyl, 250,000 people were irradiated at more than one hundred times the acceptable level; 10 percent, or twenty-five thousand people, will suffer some form of cancer in the years to come. Nuclear fallout has been detected more than 1,250 miles away from the power station; this radiation's effect on human health is still not known.

Ultraviolet Rays

Cancers of the skin (melanoma, basocellular, and squamous) are more frequent among people who work outdoors and who are exposed to the sun's ultraviolet rays for long periods of time. The frequency of skin cancers increases among individuals with fair skin and decreases among those with dark skin.

The increase in ultraviolet rays due to the destruction of the ozone layer by chlorofluorocarbons (a substance contained in refrigerators and air conditioners) translates into a growing number of cases of skin cancer.

Genetic Predisposition

We know very little about the role of each individual's genetic predisposition in the development of cancer. Sometimes, several members of the same family are stricken with cancer, either of the same type or of very different types, particularly breast cancer, sarcoma, and leukemia. However, the genetic link between these individuals is unknown.

Some cancers are described as hereditary since they can be passed from generation to generation; this is the case with a form of retinoblastoma associated with osteosarcoma, familial polyposis (a disease where a number of polyps are found in the intestine) associated with colon cancer, and certain cancers of the skin and the glandular system.

The Role of Our Natural Defense System

Studies tend to demonstrate that the human body has appropriate defense mechanisms to fight cancer. Thus, in the course of a lifetime, each individual can develop certain malignant cells, but natural mechanisms have the ability to destroy them before they become too high in number.

We have at least two barriers to defend us against cancer: the first is a mechanism to repair genes, referred to as repair enzymes, and the second is our immune system.

Repair Enzymes

This is the mechanism each cell in our body has to recognize and repair the breaks and mutations in the DNA chain. Therefore, the mechanism prevents the formation of genes that have a cancerous potential (oncogenes).

The Immune System

Not only does our immune system defend us against infections and foreign bodies, it also plays a role in defending us against the formation and progression of cancers.

This hypothesis is corroborated by certain observations; for example, leukemia patients treated through bone marrow transplants and showing graft versus host reactions (see "The GVH Reaction" in Chapter 5) run a lower risk of leukemia recurrence. The defense system, hyperreactive during the graft versus host reaction, attacks the residual leukemic cells that were not destroyed at the time of the transplant; this reaction is known as graft versus leukemia (GVL).

The recent discovery of hormones manufactured by our bodies and used to reinforce the defense system against infections, foreign bodies, and certain types of cancers has made it possible to develop new forms of cancer treatment. These drugs, natural derivatives of our bodies, are interferon (taken by patients suffering from chronic granular leukemia and hairy cell leukemia) and interleukin (used in the treatment of melanoma and certain other cancers).

Conversely, when the immune system is weakened, either by immunosuppressive drugs or by infections (such as AIDS) or congenital diseases (variable common immunodeficiency, Bruton's disease, etc.), there is an increase in the frequency of lymphoma, leukemia, sarcoma, and skin cancers.

We have long known that lymphocyte-type white cells tend to

recognize certain malignant tumors and attack them innately. Researchers with Dr. Rosenberg's team have succeeded in isolating these lymphocytes and, thanks to natural hormones (see "Gene Therapy" in Chapter 5), making them grow in very large numbers under laboratory conditions. Subsequently, these lymphocytes are reintroduced into the patient's system. Results are encouraging since the use of the lymphocytes shows a decrease in, and even a complete elimination of, tumors among patients suffering from cancers of the skin (melanoma) and kidney.

Psychological and Psychosomatic Factors

These factors undoubtedly play a major role in the development and evolution of a cancer. It is difficult to prove the link between psychological factors and cancer, but several observations are of particular interest to the medical world.

We know that individuals who experience stress run a greater risk of coronary disease and peptic ulcers; similarly, major bouts of depression are sometimes followed by the appearance of a malignant tumor within a few years. As Dr. G.R. Bach states in Creative Aggression: "An individual is more exposed to illness when he or she is depressed and has little or no aggressive energy." Furthermore, there are many examples of people who fall ill after the loss of a loved one.

The opposite is also true; some condemned patients, who have been told that they have only a few months to live, return to see their doctor (to the latter's amazement) several years later, to ask for a signature on a life insurance form or a driver's license application.

In Love, Medicine and Miracles, Dr. B. Siegel describes cases of "spontaneous remission," in other words, people who have experienced a remission that goes far beyond the prognosis given by physicians and that remains inexplicable using current scientific knowledge. He also points out that these people have an unwavering morale and an extraordinary love of and zest for life.

The most plausible scientific explanation to corroborate these observations would be neurohormones. It would seem that some hormones (unidentified to date) manufactured by the brain and released into the blood have a positive or negative influence on our immune system. When stimulated positively, our immune system slows down the progression of a cancer or even destroys it, which would explain cases of spontaneous remission. On the other hand, an inhibited immune system may not recognize a small colony of cells that have become cancerous, and the latter will form a cancer in a relatively short span of time.

As you can see, cancer is "complicated"; but thanks to the relentless work of researchers and the courage of many patients, several questions and hypotheses are now resolved.

Leukemias

Leukemias are cancers arising from the malignant transformation of hematopoietic (blood-forming) cells. The latter multiply endlessly, become very high in number, and invade the bone marrow and other organs such as the spleen, the liver, the lungs, and at times, the brain. The cancerous cells prevent healthy cells from multiplying and doing their respective jobs in organs.

Leukemia Classification

Doctors classify leukemias according to the evolution of the disease, whether acute or chronic, and according to the type of blood-forming cells (myelogenous or lymphocytic).

Classification According to the Evolution of the Disease

There are two categories of leukemia based on the severity of the illness they cause:

- Chronic leukemias, which are usually less aggressive. The cancer cells or malignant cells divide slowly and sometimes experience periods of remission extending over several months, when no treatment is necessary. Chronic leukemias can easily be treated at home, through chemotherapy drugs in pill form; in general, they cause few symptoms and patients can live entirely as they usually do. Life expectancy often extends to several years.
- Acute leukemias are more aggressive. The malignant cells (called blasts) of these leukemias divide rapidly and endlessly. Within a few weeks, several organs are affected and patients present a number of symptoms. An intensive chemotherapy treatment must be begun in a hospital within a very short period of time.

Classification According to the Type of White Cells Affected

In the blood, there are two main types of white cells: lymphocytes and granulocytes (also called polynuclear cells). We use the term lymphocytic leukemias when lymphocytes are affected, and the term myelogenous leukemias when granulocyte or polynuclear cells have become cancerous. Note: Some doctors use the term granulocytic in the place of myelogenous. Both refer to the same type of leukemia.

By linking the two major families of white cells to malignancy criteria, we obtain four types of leukemia:

1. Chronic lymphocytic leukemia (CLL)
2. Chronic myelogenous leukemia (CML)
3. Acute lymphoblastic leukemia (ALL)
4. Acute myeloblastic leukemia (AML)

    (Note that acute myeloblastic leukemias are sometimes referred to as acute nonlymphoblastic leukemias. A rare form of chronic leukemia known as hairy cell leukemia will also be examined in this chapter.)

Leukemias are also classified according to other scientific criteria, such as their microscopic morphology, their ability to absorb certain dyes (histochemistry), the presence of certain antigens on the surface of their membrane (immunology), and the presence of changes in their genes (cytogenetics). These classifications, crucial for the hematologist, are not examined in this book; they are much too complex and are not necessary for your comprehension of the subject at hand.

Chronic Leukemias

Chronic Lymphocytic Leukemia (CLL)
See Color Plate No. 6

Cancer of the white cells in the lymphocyte family mainly affects people who are approximately sixty years old. It is twice as common in men as in women and constitutes 25 percent of adult leukemia cases.

Symptoms of the Disease
CLL is often discovered by chance; a patient comes in for a routine examination and the doctor detects swelling of a lymph node and spleen. Sometimes the patient may complain of weight loss, fever, and excessive sweating at night.

Lymphocytes proliferate slowly and invade the lymph nodes, the spleen, and the liver; these organs progressively increase in size, but this enlargement is not painful. Bone marrow is affected progressively as well, and there is a slow decrease in the number of healthy white cells. Sinus and lung infections are frequent, and sometimes anemia and bruising are discovered as well.

Treatment

Treatment consists of taking chemotherapy pills (chlorambucil or cyclophosphamide) that have few side effects; at the slightest sign of sinusitis or pneumonia, the doctor will prescribe antibiotics or immunoglobulin injections. Recent studies show that stronger chemotherapies (fludarabine) used as a primary agent lead to good results as soon as the disease is diagnosed.

The Prognosis

On average, patients survive for seven years, and some live for more than fifteen years with a very good quality of life. Studies have shown that, at the time of diagnosis, if the patient suffers from anemia (less than 100 grams/L) or a decrease in the number of platelets (less than 100,000/cubic mm), or both, in general he or she will live for less than two years.

Chronic Myelogenous Leukemia (CML)
See Color Plates Nos. 3 and 4.

Cancer of the white cell in the myelogenous family is more common among men than women; the average age of patients is forty-five, but the disease can be found in younger adults as well. CML accounts for approximately 15 percent of adult leukemia cases.

The causes of CML are unknown. Certain factors, such as exposure to high-energy radiation (atomic bombs, accidents at nuclear power stations), increase the risk by fifty times. Similarly, researchers believe that certain chemical substances increase the incidence of CML; however, this cannot be scientifically proven. Such substances include benzene derivatives (paint, solvents), insecticides, pesticides, and dyes. Some anticancer drugs used jointly with radiotherapy (for example, in the treatment of lymphoma) can increase the incidence of CML several years after the treatment.

The cancerous cells of CML present a particularity of the genes in their nucleus: the leukemic cells are carriers of a mutation. For reasons that remain unknown, genes are transposed between two normal chromosomes and the result is an abnormal chromosome, easily identifiable under the microscope and known as the Philadelphia chromosome in honor of the city where it was discovered.

For a number of years, doctors were baffled by the role of the Philadelphia chromosome in CML. Recently, researchers discovered the presence of an oncogene (c-abl) on the chromosome; the oncogene seems to play a key role in the transformation of leukemic cells. The Philadelphia chromosome is present in 90 percent of patients suffering from CML; among the 10 percent who do not have this chromosome, the evolution of the disease is more violent and unpredictable.

Symptoms of the Disease

CML is often discovered in the course of a routine medical examination during which the doctor detects an increase in the number of granulocytic (polynuclear)-type white cells.

The disease can manifest itself in fatigue, heaviness in the left side of the abdomen (caused by an increase in the size of the spleen), soreness in the bones, and excessive sweating at night. More rarely, patients will complain of pains in the left side of their bodies (caused by blood circulation problems within the spleen) or will indicate that they bruise easily (caused by abnormalities in platelets). The increased uric acid produced by leukemic cells can cause kidney stones or gout. Sometimes, the leukemic cells infiltrate the central nervous system, which results in headaches and back pain. When these symptoms occur, additional diagnostic tests are needed: computerized tomography and lumbar puncture.

By palpation, the doctor will discover that the spleen and the liver have increased in size. The cellular count will reveal that the number of white cells is very high, often going beyond 100,000 per cubic millimeter (the norm being 5,000 to 10,000 per cubic millimeter). The patient sometimes suffers from anemia, and the number of platelets has decreased.

During the first two years, the evolution of CML is generally very stable; this period is the "chronic phase." Subsequently, cells become progressively resistant to treatment, and at this point the doctor must increase or modify the chemotherapies; the patient has reached the "accelerated phase." The next phase is known as the "blastic phase." At this point, the leukemia has the same characteristics as an acute leukemia. A bone biopsy and bone marrow puncture are vital to enable the doctor to establish a diagnosis and to identify the phase of the disease.

Treatment

Throughout the illness, the doctor will monitor its evolution. He or she will use physical examinations, blood tests, and bone marrow puncture on a periodic basis, since the treatment of CML is closely linked to the disease's phase.

Treatment of Patients in the Chronic Phase

If the white cell count is lower than 50,000 per cubic millimeter and if the size of the spleen is acceptable, there will be no treatment; the doctor will reevaluate the patient's condition regularly. If the white cell count is higher than 50,000 per cubic millimeter or if the spleen has increased in size, or both, treatment will consist of chemotherapy pills (bulsulfan, hydroxyurea) to be taken in small doses and periodically (for a few weeks at a time). Interferon also may be used.

Interferon (see "Immunotherapy" in Chapter 5) is a natural biological substance that increases the work done by our immune systems; it is administered daily, in small injections under the skin. In certain instances, treatment with interferon results in complete remission of the disease (normalization of the white cell count and disappearance of cells carrying the Philadelphia chromosome in the bone marrow).

New biological substances are currently under study (gamma interferon), but it is too early to predict the effect these drugs will have on the survival of patients.

Treatment of Patients in the Accelerated Phase
Treatment consists of bulsulfan and hydroxyurea administered in doses that are higher than those used in the chronic phase.

Treatment of Patients in the Blastic Phase
Treatment consists of intravenous chemotherapy based on treatment programs similar to those applied in cases of acute myelogenous leukemia. If the central nervous system has been infiltrated, radiotherapy or intrarachidian chemotherapy is used.

All these treatments are coupled with a drug (allopurinol) that prevents an excessive increase in the level of uric acid, which can damage the kidneys and cause gout.

Bone Marrow Transplants
An allogenic (with a donor who is related or unrelated to the patient) bone marrow transplant is the most effective treatment leading to the long-term cure of patients (for more details on bone marrow transplantation, see Chapter 5).

Transplants Involving Patients in the Chronic Phase Doctors prefer to proceed with a transplant within the first twelve months of diagnosis. There is no urgency for a transplant when the patient is in the chronic phase, because this phase is stable over the course of the first two years. During periodic examinations, if the doctor observes warning signs that the disease is accelerating, he or she will begin preliminary transplant procedures.

For patients who have received a transplant in the chronic phase, the rate of survival at the five-year mark is 70 percent.

Note that studies currently underway seem to show that autograft could be effective for patients who do not have a donor, although results are very fragmentary at the moment.

Transplants Involving Patients in the Accelerated or Blastic Phase The transplant must be done as soon as possible, because the disease evolves rapidly and the transplant success rate decreases as the disease progresses. When the patient is in the blastic phase, the disease must be brought into remission before the transplant can be done.

For patients who receive a transplant in the accelerated phase, the rate of survival at the five-year mark is 40 percent; it drops to 15 percent for patients in the blastic phase.

Rate of Survival, at the Five-year Mark, of Patients Suffering from CML, after a Bone Marrow Transplant

Transplant in chronic phase	70% survival
Transplant in accelerated phase	40% survival
Transplant in chronic phase	15% survival

The Prognosis
In cases where a bone marrow transplant is not possible, the average survival of patients is three to five years. However, many patients have survived for more than eight years.

Hairy Cell Leukemia
See Color Plate No. 5.

Hairy cell leukemia, also called leukemic reticuloendotheliosis, is a chronic leukemia affecting the lymphocytes. It gets its name from the fact that its leukemic cells have long filiform extensions that look like hair when examined under a microscope. Hairy cell leukemia affects men four times more often than it does women. The average age of patients is fifty. The cause of this leukemia is unknown.

Symptoms of the Disease
Hairy cell leukemia is a chronic leukemia that tends to infiltrate the bone marrow, the liver, and the spleen. The clinical manifestations of

109

the disease are the results of these infiltrations: patients complain of fatigue (caused by anemia) and are sensitive to a number of infections of the respiratory system (sinusitis, bronchitis, and pneumonia), caused by a decrease in the number of white cells. Upon physical examination, the doctor will discover that the liver and spleen have increased in size.

Unlike what occurs in the other chronic leukemias, in this instance the cell count shows a decrease in white and red cells, and platelets. The decrease in the number of blood cells is caused by the infiltration of the bone marrow by leukemic cells and by the accumulation of fibers (reticular fiber) that prevent the multiplication of healthy cells in the marrow.

A bone biopsy and bone marrow puncture are vital to enable the doctor to establish a diagnosis. The infiltration of the marrow sometimes makes the bone marrow puncture procedure difficult (dryness at the puncture site); in such cases, the diagnosis will be based on the biopsy.

Treatment

A splenectomy, or removal of the spleen, is practiced rarely (less than 10 percent of cases), and only if the spleen is very significantly enlarged. Two very effective drugs now make it possible to obtain a complete remission while avoiding splenectomy; they are interferon and 2-chlorodeoxyadenosine (2-CdA).

Interferon, discussed earlier, has a remarkable effect on hairy cell leukemia: after a few weeks of treatment, the blood cell count returns to normal and the infiltration of the bone marrow by leukemic cells decreases. According to some studies, interferon is more effective than splenectomy in patients showing a high degree of infiltration of the marrow when the disease is diagnosed, and is considered the primary form of treatment. It is administered daily in small injections under the skin. The other drug available, 2-chlorodeoxyadenosine, is also very effective; in some patients, its use in small doses can sometimes result in complete remission of the disease.

An allogenic bone marrow transplant is very effective for patients for whom drug treatments or a splenectomy have proven unsuccessful.

Prognosis

After a splenectomy, several patients have undergone remissions that have lasted for a number of years. The advent of new drugs, such as interferon, will result in a significant increase in the survival rate.

Acute Leukemias
See Color Plates Nos. 8 and 9.

Acute leukemias in adults are cancers that affect the white cells. The malignant proliferation of these cells is characterized by the formation of cancerous cells known as blasts. Blasts multiply very rapidly and tend to infiltrate many organs, which explains the very malignant potential of acute leukemias. Acute leukemias account for 50 percent of all leukemia cases in adults. They are slightly more common in men than in women.

Classification of Acute Leukemias

Blasts are young cells that multiply very rapidly and that never acquire the characteristics of normal white cells. Blasts derive from one of the two main families of white cells: lymphocytes or granulocytes. It is possible to identify their origin by viewing them through a microscope. Those from the lymphocyte family are called lymphoblasts; those from the granulocyte family are called myeloblasts. Consequently, there are two types of acute leukemias: acute lymphoblastic leukemia and acute myeloblastic leukemia. As previously mentioned, some authors refer to acute myeloblastic leukemia (AML) as acute nonlymphoblastic leukemia (ANLL) or acute granuloblastic leukemia (AGL).

The two main categories of acute leukemias can be subdivided into several subcategories, depending on the microscopic form of their blasts and their ability to absorb dyes. Thus, acute lymphoblastic leukemias are subdivided into three categories: L1, L2, and L3; acute myeloblastic leukemias are divided into seven categories: M1 to M7.

These leukemias can also be classified according to their immunological criteria (the antigens on the surface of the blasts) and cytogenetics (the abnormalities in chromosomes); all of these categories are useful for doctors when choosing a treatment program.

Factors Linked to Acute Leukemias

The following factors are not the causes of acute leukemias, but they are said to be "linked" because they increase the risk of contracting a form of the disease.

The mechanisms that result in the leukemic transformation of cells are unknown; however, the recent discovery of abnormal genes linked to cancers opens new horizons for research (see "Gene Therapy" in Chapter 5). It is possible that these factors modify the genes of healthy cells, which then become leukemic.

Ionizing Radiation
Individuals exposed to high-energy (atomic) radiation run the risk of contracting acute leukemias for twenty-five years following the exposure.

Viruses
Many retrovirus-type viruses are known to cause leukemia in mice, cats, monkeys, chickens, and cows. In humans, researchers recently identified a retrovirus, called HTLV-1 (human T cell leukemia virus), present in the leukemic cells of one type of acute lymphoblastic leukemia that has been diagnosed in patients in Japan, South Africa, and the Caribbean.

Chemical Agents
Exposure to products derived from benzene (used to manufacture paint and solvents) and to some drugs (chloramphenicol, phenylbutazone,

I
Normal blood

This photo shows the different cells that compose normal blood:

A) red cells
B) platelets
C) white cell (polynuclear type)
D) white cell (lymphocyte or granulocyte type)
E) fluid phase: plasma

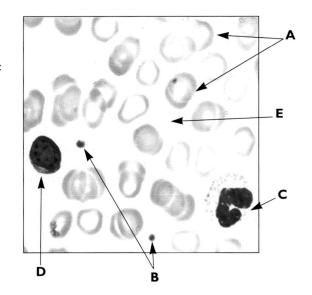

2
Normal bone marrow

Bone marrow is composed of a high number of stem cells (A), among which are found fatty cells (B) and blood cells (C).

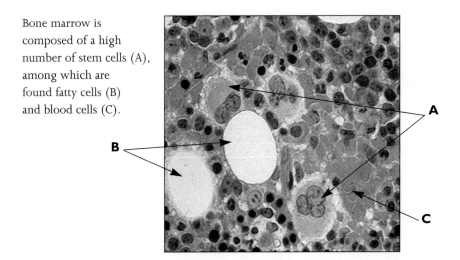

These photos show normal blood and bone marrow; they are useful for purposes of comparison with the photos on the following pages, which show the effects of various diseases.

3

Blood affected by chronic granulocytic leukemia

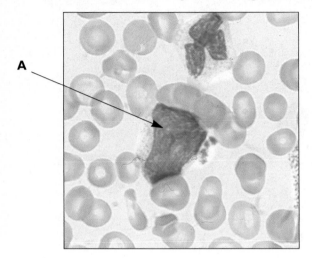

A

Note the appearance of the large white corpuscle (A), which is a cancerous cell known as a myeloblast, and is typical of this type of leukemia.

4

Bone marrow affected by chronic granulocytic leukemia

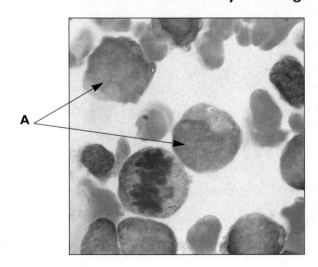

A

This bone marrow lacks normal stem cells. Note the presence of a number of myeloblasts (cancerous cells) (A).

5

Blood affected by hairy cell leukemia

In this type of leukemia, the white cells are lymphocytes with long filaments that give them a hairy appearance (A).

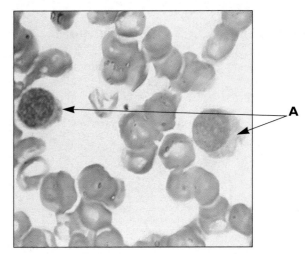

A

Chronic lymphocytic leukemia

Note the high number of white corpuscles of the lymphocyte type (A) among the red corpuscles (B).

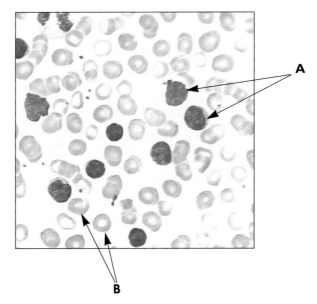

A

B

7

Bone marrow affected by aplasia or fibrosis

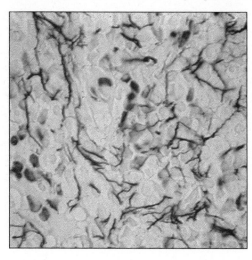

Note the lack of stem cells, which have been replaced by reticular fiber or fibrosis (in green). The marrow is unable to manufacture blood.

8

Bone marrow affected by acute myeloblastic leukemia

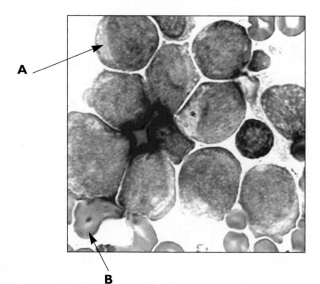

A

B

Note the very high number of cancerous cells of the myelobast type (A) that invade the bone marrow. Simultaneously, there is a major decrease in all stem cells and red cells (B).

9

Bone marrow affected by acute lymphoblastic leukemia

Note the high number of lymphoblast type cells (A) and the decrease in red cells (B) and stem cells.

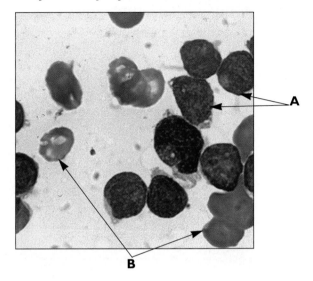

A

B

Microscopic transection of a normal lymph node

Note the mass of cells known as follicles (A). The follicles are sites where lymphocytes multiply in response to an exterior stimulus such as a viral infection.

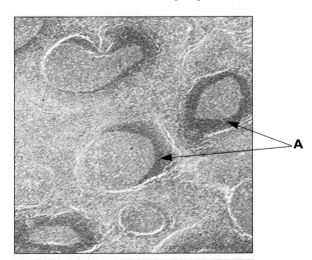

A

This photo is useful for purposes of comparison with Color Plates 11 and 12, which show lymphomas.

11
Microscopic transection of a lymph node affected by non-Hodgkin lymphoma

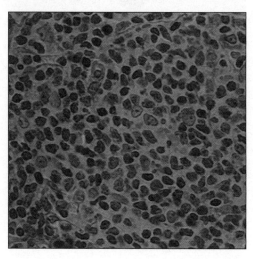

In this photo, a follicle has been invaded by cancerous lymphocytes. The lymphocyte invasion results in a swelling of the lymph nodes.

12
Microscopic transection of a lymph node affected by Hodgkin's lymphoma

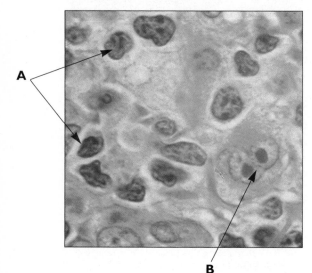

A

B

Note the disappearance of normal lymphocyte follicles caused by the invasion of numerous cancerous lymphocytes (A). Hodgkin's lymphoma is characterized by the presence of cells known as Reed-Sternberg cells (B). The origin and the role of these cells in disease is unknown.

13

Microscopic view of bone marrow affected by myeloma

The bone marrow is invaded by cancerous cells of the myelomatic type (A), which are characteristic of myeloma.

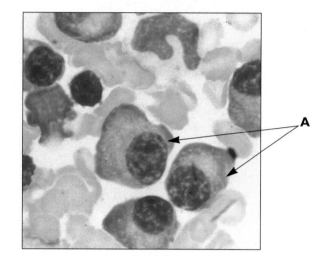

A

Microscopic view of a drop of blood taken from a child suffering from sickle cell anemia

This form of hereditary disease, called sickle cell anemia, is characterized by a decrease in the red corpuscles, which take on a sickle shape.

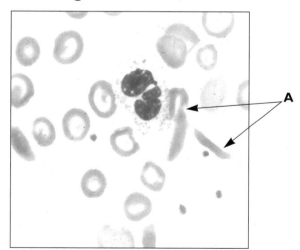

A

15

Bone marrow affected by a metastasis

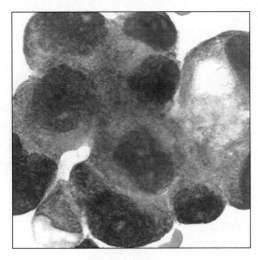

This photo shows the multiplication of cancerous cells resulting from lung cancer. The cells invade the bone marrow and prevent the formation of normal blood.

16

Microscopic view of bone marrow affected by the myelodysplasic syndrome or preleukemia

A

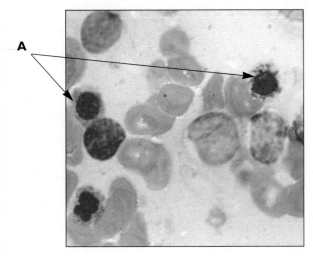

This photo of bone marrow affected by the myelodysplasic syndrome shows the presence of cancerous cells whose edges form a type of blue-colored ring or crown (A). These cells are known as ring sideroblasts and their number determines the gravity and progression of the disease.

alkylating agents) has been recognized as a factor that can increase the risk of acute myeloblastic leukemia.

Symptoms of Acute Leukemias

Acute leukemias evolve very rapidly, because blasts infiltrate the bone marrow and prevent healthy cells from multiplying. The symptoms presented by patients are linked to the infiltration of various organs; thus, when the bone marrow is affected, the result is anemia, hemorrhages, and infections. Almost all organs can be infiltrated by leukemic cells, but some, such as the central nervous system, the liver, the spleen, and the lymph nodes, are affected more frequently.

Symptoms Caused by Infiltration of the Bone Marrow

Anemia
The decrease in the number of red cells causes fatigue, pallor, shortness of breath, and headaches.

Hemorrhages
The decrease in the number of platelets (less than twenty thousand per cubic millimeter) leads to an increase in all types of bleeding. The most frequent are bruising, heavy menstruation, gums that bleed when teeth are brushed or extracted, and nosebleeds.

Acute myeloblastic leukemias (type M3, in particular) lead to more hemorrhages than do acute lymphoblastic leukemias.

Infections
Even if there is a high number of leukemic cells in the blood, note that these malignant cells are immature and unable to protect the organism against infections. Patients will be more sensitive to infections of the respiratory system, the skin, the kidneys, and the bladder.

Bone Pain

Infiltration of the bones causes bone pain in more than 25 percent of patients suffering from acute leukemias.

Symptoms Caused by Infiltration of Other Organs

The Central Nervous System

The infiltration of this organ can be completely symptom-free or it can cause various symptoms, ranging from headaches, nausea, and vomiting to paralysis of certain parts of the body.

Usually, a lumbar puncture is used to evaluate the presence of leukemic cells.

Other Organs

The liver, the spleen, and the lymph nodes often increase in size. More rarely, acute myeloblastic leukemia infiltrates the skin and forms a greenish-colored tumor known as a chloroma. Acute lymphoblastic leukemia often attacks the testicles, especially during a recurrence.

Diagnosis

A complete cell count usually indicates the presence of anemia and a decrease in the number of platelets, while the number of white cells may have increased, remained normal, or decreased. Often, large quantities of blasts are found in the blood.

Bone marrow puncture and biopsy are vital for microscopic examination and to establish a diagnosis.

Electrolyte elements (potassium, sodium, calcium, phosphorus) in the blood can sometimes be affected, and certain products originating in leukemic cells, such as uric acid, can damage the kidneys.

Treatment of Acute Leukemias in Adults

Only a few years ago, patients suffering from acute leukemias always died within a short time span. Recent treatments using multiple chemotherapy agents led to remission (a normalization of all blood and bone marrow tests as well as the patient's symptoms and physical examination) in the majority of cases.

Initial treatment consists of correcting the metabolic abnormalities (potassium, sodium, calcium, phosphorus, uric acid), anemia, hemorrhages, and infections; this stage is the support treatment and it usually takes twenty-four to forty-eight hours.

Any patient in this situation should read Chapter 5.

Treatment of Acute Lymphoblastic Leukemias in Adults
The treatment includes four phases: induction of remission, prophylactic treatment of the central nervous system, maintenance treatment (see Chapter 5), and if necessary, bone marrow transplant.

Induction of Remission
The combination of two or more chemotherapeutic agents (prednisone, vincristine, L-asparaginase, doxorubicine, or daunorubicine) results in remission in more than 90 percent of patients aged fifteen to thirty years old and in 60 to 70 percent of those over thirty.

Remission induction treatment requires hospitalization over a period of a few weeks.

Prophylactic Treatment of the Central Nervous System
Acute lymphoblastic leukemia often penetrates the central nervous system.

Preventive treatment through radiotherapy and the injection of chemotherapy (methotrexate) in the cerebrospinal fluid decreases recurrences in this location. This treatment usually starts after the remission induction treatment.

Maintenance Treatment

A few chemotherapy agents are administered every four or six weeks over a period of several months (up to one to three years), depending on the treatment program used (see Chapter 5).

Recurrences

If the leukemia reappears, the doctor must proceed with a second remission induction treatment.

Bone Marrow Transplant

Some studies favor a bone marrow transplant in all adult patients after a first remission; others reserve it for those who suffer from high-risk leukemias (involving difficulty in inducing remission) and for patients who have had a recurrence and who experience a second remission.

Both types of bone marrow transplant can be effective: a graft with a compatible donor, or when no donor is available, an autograft with depletion of cancerous cells. Bone marrow transplant with a donor presents a cure rate of 60 percent; autograft has a cure rate of 40 to 50 percent.

Treatment of Acute Myeloblastic Leukemias

The treatment includes three phases: induction of remission, consolidation treatment, and bone marrow transplant.

Induction of Remission

Thanks to new chemotherapy treatment programs making joint use of various drugs such as cytosine arabinoside and anthracyclines, remission induction is possible in more than 60 to 80 percent of patients.

Consolidation Treatment

Despite the progress made in the area of remission induction, remission usually lasts only a few months if no other treatment is given. Therefore, two or three more cycles of "consolidation" chemotherapy are usually given to prolong remission duration. The overall cure rate with this approach is slightly above 20 percent.

Bone Marrow Transplant

This form of treatment offers the best cure rate; given the high level of recurrence of AML, bone marrow transplants are done after the first remission.

The success rate of transplants with compatible donors is 60 percent. The recent development of the autograft with selective depletion of cancerous cells leads to cure rates in the order of 45 percent for patients for whom no compatible donor can be found.

Leukemias in Children

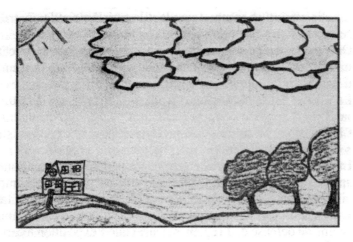

This drawing was given to me by a little girl who had just finished two years of intensive treatments against an acute form of leukemia.

Despite its very simple lines, it expresses a victory: The sun is peeking out of a corner as huge black clouds seem to be traveling away. Three healthy trees are perched on a hill overlooking endless fields. A multi-windowed house is a perfect vantage point on the beautiful surroundings.

Nathalie went on to become a tall and beautiful young girl—she has an endearing smile, the very same smile that the black clouds of illness chased away seven years ago. Today, her smile brings a blush to the face of just about every boy at her school.

Nathalie still loves to tease her two younger brothers.

Under a cascade of curls, her huge eyes seem to have a lot to say; they never seem to focus on any one thing for very long—there are too many things to look at.

And after all these years, Nathalie's favorite color is still green, the symbol of hope.

Acute leukemias are the most common forms of leukemia found in children under fifteen years of age. The incidence of the disease is highest between one and five years, and it peaks during the third and fourth year of a child's life. It is estimated that the risk of a child contracting leukemia during the first fifteen years of life is approximately one in twenty-four thousand.

Risk is an epidemiological indicator that evaluates the probability of contracting a given disease. It is a useful indicator in identifying subjects or groups exposed to certain situations or factors. Risk value is determined based on observations that apply to select groups. Using these observations, doctors compare groups of children to determine whether family-related or genetic factors, the presence of joint disease weakening the body's defense system, and exposure to certain drugs and environmental factors actually increase the risk of contracting leukemia.

This specific risk value is then compared to the risk that characterizes the general population. The closer the risk value comes to the risk in the general population, the less chance there is that the subject could contract a given disease. To better understand risk value, consider the example of children exposed to high levels of atomic radiation as the result of an accident at a nuclear power station. After exposure, the risk of leukemia would be approximately one in sixty over a period of twelve years; thus, in each group of sixty children exposed to the radiation, one child will contract leukemia within twelve years of the exposure. As you can see, for children exposed to radiation, the risk of contracting leukemia is enormous—in the general population, the risk is only one child in twenty-four thousand.

Family-related and Genetic Factors

- The risk for the brothers and sisters of a leukemic child: There is virtually no increase in the risk for the brothers and sisters of a child who has contracted leukemia. The risk is comparable to the risk that exists in the general population.
- The risk for fraternal twins: It is comparable to the risk for sisters and brothers and, therefore, for the population in general.
- The risk for identical twins: The risk for a child whose identical twin has contracted leukemia is one in eight before the age of ten. This risk is staggering! We cannot explain the reasons underlying this observation, but we believe that genetic factors play a part in increasing the risk in these children. Since identical twins have identical genes, researchers hypothesize that fetal oncogenes cause leukemia among very young children; others believe that these children have genes that predispose them to leukemia, making them more sensitive to certain risk factors (environmental factors, viruses, etc.). However, note that identical twins who are both healthy have no greater risk of contracting leukemia than does the general population.
- The risk related to maternal or paternal factors: No direct link has been established between certain diseases affecting parents and the development of leukemia in children. When treating pregnant women, doctors avoid drugs known to affect the bone marrow and X-rays, which increase the risk of leukemia among children (one in sixteen thousand compared to one in twenty-four thousand in the general population). Smoking during pregnancy seems to significantly increase the risk of leukemia in children.

119

Environmental Factors

Some studies have shown that children whose parents work in industries where they come into regular contact with pesticides, chlorinated solvents, and hydrocarbons, and whose parents work in the aerospace industry have significantly greater incidence rates of leukemia. The environmental factors involved in the development of cancer in adults, such as drugs (alkylating agents) and benzene-based solvents, have the same effects in children. Studies also tend to show that children who live in areas where underground water tables contain radium or who live in houses located near high-voltage electric power lines could have a higher risk of contracting leukemia.

However, comparative studies have failed to corroborate these findings. Therefore, it would be wrong to draw conclusions too hastily since epidemiological studies are never entirely reliable and several intrinsic problems may provide biased final results. As long as our scientific facts on leukemia are not solid, we need other comparative studies before we can conclude that a given environmental factor has an actual potential to cause leukemia.

Related Diseases Increasing the Risk of Leukemia

Several congenital diseases are linked to an increase in leukemia rates. These include trisomy (Down's syndrome) and diseases affecting the immune system, such as Fanconi's anemia, Wiskott-Aldrich syndrome, and combined severe immunodeficiency (these diseases are discussed in the section entitled "Congenital Diseases of the Blood System"—see pages 149–55).

The frequency of leukemia is slightly higher among children who have been treated for another form of cancer; these leukemias are described as secondary and they occur more frequently after a treatment program combining chemotherapy and radiotherapy. Thus, the type of cancer treated previously has no real impact in the development of secondary leukemia. To decrease the risk of secondary leukemia, doctors now avoid combining radiotherapy and chemotherapy in a single treatment program.

The Causes of Leukemia in Children

The development of leukemia in children involves several factors that interact and that are genetic, hormonal, immunological, and environmental in nature. On the basis of findings to date, researchers presume that the disturbance causing a cell to become cancerous occurs in the genes (a portion of the DNA chain). These defective genes, oncogenes, transmit erroneous messages to the cell, including the message to multiply nonstop.

The recent discovery of oncogenes is a major step forward in cancer research; furthermore, it opens many avenues in the development of new treatments (see pages 87–89).

Symptoms of Leukemia in Children

Acute lymphoblastic leukemia accounts for more than 85 percent of leukemia cases in children; the remaining 15 percent is composed of acute leukemias of the myeloblastic type and, very rarely, chronic myelogenous leukemias (less than 1 percent).

Symptoms of acute leukemia vary from child to child. In general, they appear six to eight weeks before the parents consult a physician and a diagnosis is made, and they are not specific to the disease. The child is fatigued, has less energy than usual, and sometimes complains of joint, muscle, and bone pain. He or she is more susceptible to infections such as otitis, bronchitis, and pneumonia.

The decrease in the number of red cells will result in anemia, which causes pallor, fatigue, and shortness of breath. The decrease in the number of platelets increases the risk of bleeding, although it will usually be minor: excessive bleeding from the gums when brushing the teeth, bruising, or nose bleeds. These types of bleeding rarely endanger a child's life.

During the physical examination, the doctor will notice that the child is pale and irritable or that the lymph nodes, the liver, or the spleen have increased in size. Among boys, the testicles may also increase in size.

At times, leukemic cells may infiltrate the skin, marking it with bruiselike blotches that do not seem to heal.

The Risk of Leukemia among Certain Select Groups of Children

Select groups	Risk of contracting leukemia
Normal children (general population)	1 in 24,000 before the age of 15
Presence of leukemia in identical twins	Risk for the second twin: 1 in 8 before the age of 10
Related diseases:	
• Trisomy (Down's syndrome)	1 in 74 before the age of 10
• Congenital diseases affecting the immune system	1 in 12 before the age of 21
Exposure to certain factors	
• Nuclear radiation	Can increase the risk to 1 in 60 for 12 years following exposure
• Certain drugs (alkylating agents)	1 in 500 during the 20 years following exposure

Diagnosis
(See also Chapter 3.)

A complete cell count makes it possible to verify whether the number of white cells has decreased, is normal, or has increased. Leukemic cells (blast) present in the blood can total more than fifty thousand. In general, the number of red cells, the hemoglobin level, and the platelet level have decreased.

A biopsy and bone marrow puncture are vital in establishing a diagnosis. They are practiced on one of the posterior iliac crests or at the sternum. The biopsy and the puncture make it possible to take a sample including a large number of leukemic cells, which are then sent to a laboratory where they are examined under a microscope and submitted to a number of other tests (lymphocyte marker analysis, cytogenetics, biochemistry, etc.). These tests allow doctors to identify the type of leukemia affecting the child.

A lumbar puncture makes it possible to take a sample of several cubic centimeters of cerebrospinal liquid; leukemic cells sometimes infiltrate the liquid surrounding the brain.

Blood tests are done at the time of diagnosis and regularly thereafter to monitor blood biochemistry, which reflects the functioning of the child's organs. Special attention is paid to the functioning of the kidneys and the liver and the accumulation of products generated by leukemic cells, such as uric acid.

Permanent or temporary subcutaneous catheters (porto-caths) can be put into place in the operating room. They facilitate blood tests and make the intravenous administration of drugs pain-free.

The medical team will examine all of the organs that may be affected by the leukemia; an ultrasonography examination of the abdomen and an X-ray of the lungs will be used to detect the presence of lymph node enlargement or abnormal masses; if neurological symptoms are present, the brain will be examined using computerized tomography technology.

In children, leukemia is investigated and treated by a multidisciplinary team.

Treatment and Prognosis

The success rates of treating leukemia in children has increased steadily in the past twenty years. Today, more than 70 percent of the total number of children suffering from leukemia experience remissions lasting more than five years.

This success can be attributed to the development of more precise diagnostic techniques. In fact, there are several leukemia subtypes, and each of these subtypes is linked to a specific treatment program.

Types of Leukemia and Their Incidence in Children

Acute lymphoblastic (L1, L2, L3) (ALL)	85%
Acute myeloblastic leukemia (AML)	14%
Chronic myelogenous leukemia (CML)	less than 1%

After identifying the type of leukemia the child has contracted, the doctor must determine whether the disease's prognosis is good or poor. Using prognostic factors, doctors attempt to predict how leukemias will develop, differentiating those that will have a violent progression (in other words, those that will resist treatment and will cause a quick recurrence) from those that will respond to treatment and will not cause a recurrence. Therefore, there are favorable prognostic factors, which are most often linked to leukemias with a good prognosis, and unfavorable prognostic factors, which are frequently associated with leukemias whose prognosis is not good.

Whether the leukemic child presents favorable or unfavorable factors, there is no certitude of the evolution or the prognosis of the leukemia. These factors are merely indicators that can help the medical team make a decision on how to treat the child.

The prognosis of the child's leukemia is made using several clinical factors and laboratory tests. The main factors are age, the initial white cell count, the presence of tumorous masses (infiltration of the liver, the spleen, the lymph nodes, the testicles), the hemoglobin level, the number of platelets, and the response to remission induction chemotherapy treatment. The factors that seem to have the strongest prediction value are age, the number of white cells at diagnosis, the presence of major tumorous masses, and the response to remission induction chemotherapy (see the table below).

The Main Prognostic Factors of Acute Lymphoblastic Leukemia

Factors	More favorable	Less favorable
Age	Between 2 and 9 years old	Less than 1 year old; more than 10 years old
Initial white cell count (per cubic millimeter)	Fewer than 10,000	More than 50,000
Tumorous masses	Absence	Presence
Hemoglobin	Fewer than 8 grams/dL	More than 10 grams/dL
Number of platelets (per cubic millimeter)	Fewer than 100,000	More than 100,000
Response, after two weeks, to chemotherapy applied by bone marrow puncture	Excellent—less than 5% of blasts	Poor—more than 25% of blasts

The Specifics of Treating Children

Generally, remission induction treatment involves a combination of three or four chemotherapies; the basic drugs are prednisone and vincristine. The treatment, which requires that the child be hospitalized for a few weeks, is designed to rapidly destroy the greatest possible number of leukemic cells. At the two-week mark, a bone marrow puncture is performed to verify the treatment's effectiveness.

Intensification or consolidation treatment begins immediately after the remission induction treatment; it reduces the number of residual leukemic cells even further. Intensification treatment is particularly effective in preventing recurrences among children whose prognosis was established as poor at the time of diagnosis.

The brain is a frequent site of leukemic recurrences; before the discovery of prophylactic treatments, more than 80 percent of children experienced recurrences within the first three years of the remission induction treatment. The brain is wrapped in a envelope called the hemo-encephalic barrier, which prevents most drugs used in chemotherapy from penetrating but lets leukemic cells enter freely.

To reach these cancerous cells, the doctor injects a chemotherapy drug, most often a methotrexate, directly into the cerebrospinal fluid; this treatment is often coupled with localized radiotherapy (see "Radiotherapy" in Chapter 5). Prophylactic treatment of the nervous system usually begins after the remission induction treatment.

For children whose prognosis is good, doctors use only chemotherapy. If the prognosis is poor, several sessions of localized radiotherapy will be used to treat the central nervous system.

Prophylactic treatment of the central nervous system does have side effects; after a few weeks, close to half of the children given methotrexate and radiotherapy suffer from irritability and anorexia, somnolence, fever, nausea, vomiting, and diarrhea. In rare instances, the combination of methotrexate and radiotherapy can lead to long-term side effects in some children. The effects vary and range from minor learning problems to more severe manifestations such as a decrease in the intelligence quotient, a decrease in growth, and more rarely still, damage to certain parts of the brain.

In spite of its side effects, prophylactic treatment decreases the rate of recurrences in the central nervous system from 40 percent to less than 6 percent; it also leads to a decrease of recurrences in other parts of the body.

Researchers are working to improve prophylactic treatment programs by diminishing their side effects while maintaining their effectiveness at preventing recurrences.

Since the testicles are also a frequent site of leukemic recurrences, in some cases they may be irradiated.

Maintenance treatment is designed to prevent long-term recurrences of leukemia. It begins after the remission induction and consolidation treatments; several chemotherapies are used at intervals of two to three weeks, over a period of several months.

General Side Effects

For a description of general side effects, see "Chemotherapy" in Chapter 5. However, for children, there are also side effects on growth, as radiotherapy can damage the pituitary gland, located in the brain. This gland secretes several hormones, including the hormone that controls growth in children. If the growth hormone's level decreases because the pituitary gland is not functioning properly, growth will be slowed and the child will be smaller than a normal child. Luckily, the growth hormone is now available in the form of a drug and its use ensures that the child develops normally.

Side Effects on the Reproductive System

Boys may become sterile, because the cells that form sperm are very sensitive to leukemia treatments; however, sexual functions are completely unaffected. Generally, the sterility rate is higher when the testicles are irradiated. In the case of an adolescent, sperm may be removed before treatment and kept frozen throughout the patient's lifetime.

Among girls treated before puberty, reproductive functions can be preserved. Among young pubescent girls and female adolescents, the reproductive system seems to be much more sensitive to treatments and, therefore, the long-term infertility rate is higher.

127

A study conducted among young adults who were treated for leukemia during the 1970s shows that, out of 1,500 pregnancies, the rates of spontaneous abortion, pregnancy-related complications, and congenital malformations are identical to the rates recorded for the general population. Therefore, young girls and young boys treated for leukemia, and whose reproductive functions are intact, can have normal and healthy children.

Other Types of Malignant Blood Diseases

Aplastic Anemia
See Color Plate No. 7.

Aplastic anemia, or aplasia of the bone marrow, is a disease in which the bone marrow stops manufacturing blood cells. For reasons that remain unknown, stem cells lose their ability to multiply, leaving an empty space in the bone marrow; this empty space is filled by fatty cells. Although many cases of aplastic anemia are not malignant, in the sense of cancerous, some are considered to be "preneoplastic"; i.e., they may evolve into overt leukemia or myelodysplastic syndrome.

Although found in patients of all ages, aplastic anemia is most common in adults aged sixty and over. In children, it is linked to rare congenital diseases (Fanconi's anemia, Diamond Blackfan anemia), which will be discussed later in this chapter.

The mechanisms that cause stem cells to stop multiplying are unknown; however, several factors, including our immune system and certain other factors listed in this section, are involved in the development of aplastic anemia.

Environmental Factors

Repeated or constant exposure to certain chemical products found in solvents and paint (benzene, toluene, tetrachloride) and to pesticides and insecticides (DDT, parathion, pentachlorophenol) can increase the risk of aplastic anemia.

Nuclear radiation destroys the stem cells directly and causes aplastic anemia, especially if received in high doses.

Drugs

All chemotherapeutic agents decrease stem cell multiplication (see "Chemotherapy" in Chapter 5). In general, this side effect is linked to the dose of the drug used in the treatment and lasts only for the period of time during which the treatment is administered. As soon as treatment stops, cells behave normally again.

Unfortunately, some antibiotics, the most well known being chloramphenicol, cause irreversible aplastic anemia, even when used in very small quantities (idiosyncratic effect). In industrialized countries, this antibiotic is still used in drop and ointment form for eye infections (conjunctivitis); even in small doses, chloramphenicol can cause irreversible aplasia in one user in twenty-five thousand—a risk that seems to have been deemed acceptable! Furthermore, more extensive use of chloramphenicol is common in developing countries, where drug restrictions are lax.

Several other drugs have the rare side effects of slowing the growth of stem cells and causing aplasia; these phenomena are usually reversible and cells behave normally when administration stops or when doses are decreased. These drugs include antibiotics, antihistamines, anticonvulsants, and tranquilizers. To prevent aplastic anemia, the doctor must proceed with periodic blood analyses (complete cell counts) whenever these particular drugs are used.

Links with Certain Diseases

The link between viral hepatitis (more often Type C) and aplastic anemia is found more often in children. Hepatitis-related aplasia is more frequent among boys than girls and it develops a few months after the hepatitis.

Sometimes, and more often in children, aplasia appears a few months before leukemia.

Reversible aplasia is often concomitant to other diseases such as lupus erythematosus, rheumatoid arthritis, and some cancers (thymus). In the large majority of cases, medical control of these diseases will normalize the aplasia.

Symptoms of Aplastic Anemia

Symptoms are linked to the decrease in the three large lines of blood cells (red cells, white cells, and platelets). Generally, symptoms are insidious: patients complain of fatigue, shortness of breath, headaches, and pallor (symptoms linked to the decrease in red cells or anemia). Furthermore, the decrease in platelets leads to minor bleeding from the gums when the teeth are brushed, nosebleeds, and often, among young women, an increase in menstrual flow. The decrease in white cells leads to an increase in infections of the respiratory system (sinusitis, laryngitis, bronchitis, and pneumonia). At times, aplasia may be present in the form of hemorrhages and very severe infections, although such occurrences are very rare.

Diagnosis

A complete cell count shows a decrease in white cells, red cells, and platelets. Sometimes, early in the disease, this decrease affects only one line of blood cells.

The bone marrow puncture shows only a few stem cells and a high number of fatty cells. It is often "dry"; in other words, the doctor cannot remove even the smallest bone marrow sample, so instead will have to perform a bone biopsy.

Treatment

The first step in treatment consists of neutralizing the complications, such as infections, serious hemorrhaging, and anemia. As soon as the patient is no longer in danger, the doctor evaluates the possibility of proceeding with a bone marrow transplant. An allogenic transplant leads to a long-term cure.

If at all possible, the medical team will avoid giving the patient transfusions, except in cases involving anemia or a very low platelet count. This measure prevents graft versus host rejections (see "Bone Marrow Transplant" in Chapter 5).

If the patient cannot be given a bone marrow transplant, either because there is no compatible donor or because of contraindications (advanced age), other forms of treatment will be used. While they do not lead to a cure, they often result in a remission that lasts for several years.

1. Antilymphocytic globulins. These are antibodies directed against a certain type of white cell, the lymphocytes. These drugs, administered by injection, lead to an improvement in symptoms in the majority of patients.
2. Androgens. These drugs are derived from male hormones and are administered by injection or in the form of tablets. Androgens sometimes make it possible to improve the patient's condition and to slow the disease's progression.
3. Immunosuppressive drugs: Immunosuppressive drugs, such as cyclosporin, and corticosteroids given at high doses, often in combination.

Drugs to Avoid
A patient suffering from aplastic anemia should avoid drugs such as aspirin, which can affect the functioning of platelets, thus increasing the risk of bleeding.

Prognosis
The long-term treatment of aplasia is a bone marrow transplant with a compatible donor. In such cases, the cure rate is 60 to 70 percent. Among patients who cannot be given a transplant, the prognosis varies greatly. For unknown reasons, some patients react very well to drugs, while

others are totally resistant. Often, the doctor must test several drugs and, sometimes, must use a combination of two drugs to achieve remission.

The Myelodysplasic Syndrome or Myelodysplasia
See Color Plate No. 16.

Myelodysplasia is a cancerous disease of the bone marrow. The average age of patients suffering from this disease is fifty, but young adults can also be affected by it. This leukemia progresses slowly and, in the relative short term, tends to change into acute leukemia.

Symptoms of the Disease
Most symptoms seen in patients are linked to the infiltration of the bone marrow by malignant cells: anemia causes fatigue, pallor, and shortness of breath; the decrease in white cells results in an increase in infections (sinusitis, bronchitis, pneumonia, and others); and the decrease in platelets causes an increase in bleeding (bruising, bleeding from the gums, a heavier menstrual flow, etc.).

The bone marrow puncture is vital in establishing a diagnosis; it shows the abnormalities in stem cells and the presence of blasts, called ring sideroblasts (see the color plate). If the disease progresses toward acute leukemia, the number of blasts increases.

Treatment and Prognosis
The average survival of a patient suffering from myelodysplasic syndrome varies from eight to forty months.

Based on the microscopic study of the patient's bone marrow, doctors can predict how the disease will progress. If it shows signs of progressing toward acute leukemia, the doctors will proceed with a bone marrow transplant with a compatible donor. Currently, the allogenic transplant is the only long-term curative treatment and the success rate is in the order of fifty percent.

Thrombocythemia

This disease is characterized by an increase in the number of platelets in the blood. The average age at diagnosis is sixty, although in rare instances young adults can also contract the disease.

The causes of basic thrombocythemia are unknown. Before making a diagnosis, the doctor will eliminate all diseases that can result in an increase in the number of platelets: chronic inflammatory diseases, infections, and some specific types of cancer.

Symptoms of the Disease

Most patients are asymptomatic at the time of diagnosis. Often, the disease is discovered following a blood test that is part of a routine medical examination.

In spite of the very high number of platelets (more than 600,000 per cubic millimeter), because they have lost their ability to form blood clots, symptoms often include bleeding (bruising, bleeding from the gums or the nose, bleeding in the digestive tract).

If the number of platelets increases significantly (more than one million per cubic millimeter), the blood will become more viscous and the risk of thromboses will increase; this problem will manifest itself mainly in the small blood vessels of the hands and feet, and will cause a burning sensation.

The spleen sometimes increases in size.

Prognosis and Treatment

The prognosis for this disease is ten years, and sometimes more. Most patients will not require any form of treatment for several years.

Aspirin seems to decrease the risk of thrombosis by preventing the aggregation of the platelets.

Basic chemotherapy treatment (bulsulfan, anagrelide, hydroxyurea) in tablet form will be administered only if the number of platelets is very high and if the patient is experiencing thromboses.

Bone marrow transplant with a donor makes it possible to cure young adults who have contracted the rarer and more severe forms of the disease.

Polycythemia or Vaquez's Disease

Polycythemia is a disease whose main characteristic is an increase in the number of red cells. A malignant disorder of the stem cells in the bone marrow seems to be the origin of this disease.

Several factors lead to an increase in the number of red cells without the presence of polycythemia. These factors are linked to conditions or diseases that lower the level of oxygen in the blood: smoking combined with stress, living at high altitudes, and lung or heart diseases. Another factor is conditions of severe dehydration: among patients with severe burns, individuals suffering from severe diarrhea or excessive vomiting, in the case of certain kidney diseases (cysts) or certain benign tumors (uterine fibroma, adrenal glands) or malignant tumors (liver, ovaries, uterus).

The doctor must always look for secondary factors that cause an increase in the number of red cells; when these factors are corrected, the number of red cells will return to the normal level automatically. In cases of polycythemia, the number of red cells remains high.

The average age at diagnosis ranges between fifty-five and sixty-five; the disease rarely affects individuals in their forties. It is slightly more common among men than women.

Symptoms of the Disease

In large part, the symptoms of this disease are linked to the major increase in the number of red cells; in fact, their number becomes so high that the blood becomes more viscous, which causes problems with circulation. Concomitant symptoms vary: a sensation of heat in the hands and feet, headaches, dizziness, problems with vision, shortness of breath, and various forms of phlebitis. Other symptoms such as pruritis (itchiness), gout, and hemorrhaging also may be present.

During a physical examination, the doctor will notice that the patient has a red face and that the spleen and liver are larger than normal.

Laboratory examinations will show an increase in the number of red cells and the hemoglobin level and, at times, in the number of white cells and platelets. The calculation of the total number of red cells, using the isotopic method (nuclear medicine), always shows an increase.

Treatment and Prognosis

Treatment consists of removing five hundred cubic centimeters of blood at one time, at first once or twice a week and then monthly, to maintain the number of red cells at acceptable levels. Other forms of treatment are sometimes administered at the same time, such as chemotherapy in tablet form and in small doses (myleran, hydroxyurea) or in the form of radioactive phosphorus.

To prevent gout and pruritis, the doctor will prescribe allopurinol and cimetidine in tablet form.

The prognosis for this disease is excellent; the average survival is twelve years, but many patients have survived for twenty years, and one is still alive after thirty-five years.

Severe complications include phlebitis, myelofibrosis (see below), and, more rarely, acute leukemia, can occur.

Myelofibrosis
See Color Plate No. 7.

Myelofibrosis is a bone marrow disease that affects individuals aged fifty-five and over; it is rarely found in individuals aged forty or younger. In this disease, normal bone marrow is replaced by a compact and fibrous substance (fibrous connective tissue). It spreads within the bone and, eventually, occupies all of the space reserved for stem cells, which can no longer multiply; as a result, the blood slowly loses cells and platelets.

For most patients, doctors are unable to identify the cause of myelofibrosis, in which case it is described as primary. Occasionally, it is linked to other malignant diseases such as leukemia, lymphoma, and other types of cancer, to inflammatory diseases, and, more rarely, to chronic infections (tuberculosis). The doctor will always look for secondary causes before making a final diagnosis.

Symptoms of the Disease

At the outset, the disease is often insidious and symptoms reflect the degree to which the bone marrow is affected: anemia (fatigue, pallor, and shortness of breath) and a decrease in the number of platelets, which can predispose the patient to hemorrhaging. Generally, the number of white cells is the same, which ensures adequate protection against infections. The spleen is swollen and causes a sensation of heaviness and sometimes pain in the left side of the body.

When the disease has progressed for a few years, the liver and heart can show signs of failure.

Bone marrow puncture is difficult to do and taking a cell sample may not be possible; such punctures are known as blank or dry. A bone biopsy is vital in establishing a diagnosis: the bone is hard and it contains a very significant amount of fibrous connective tissue and very few stem cells.

Treatment and Prognosis

Unfortunately, there is no specific treatment for this disease. Hormone-based treatments (androgens) sometimes help to control the anemia temporarily. Some studies report isolated cases in which a bone marrow transplant has proven to be successful.

The disease progresses slowly. Life expectancy is eight to ten years. Patients are monitored regularly by the doctor, who seeks to prevent and treat complications.

For unknown reasons, this disease sometimes progresses into acute leukemia.

Malignant Diseases of the Immune System
See Color Plates Nos. 10, 11, and 12.

Lymphomas

Lymphomas, cancers that affect the lymph nodes (see Chapter 2), are divided into two types: non-Hodgkin lymphoma and Hodgkin's lymphoma. The name comes from Thomas Hodgkin, who in 1832 was the first to describe the disease.

Today, the microscopic study of tissues taken from lymphomatic nodes makes it possible to differentiate between these two types of lymphomas and to establish a precise diagnosis, vital for the doctor to prescribe an appropriate treatment.

Within the lymph nodes affected by non-Hodgkin lymphoma, there is an infiltration of small lymphocytic-type, cancerous white cells. In cases of Hodgkin's lymphoma, large cancerous cells known as Reed-Sternberg cells have infiltrated the nodes.

Non-Hodgkin lymphomas affect people of all ages, but are more common among men than women. The incidence of the disease is higher in certain parts of the world, such as Central Africa, the West Indies, and Japan, and may be the result of viral infections; in fact, the presence of the mononucleosis virus (Epstein-Barr virus) is noted among Africans, and the presence of the ATL (adult T lymphoma) virus is seen among Japanese and West Indian patients.

A chronic weakening of the immune system can also increase the incidence of non-Hodgkin lymphomas. Thus, among children suffering from certain rare congenital diseases that weaken the immune system, we observe an increase in the number of non-Hodgkin lymphomas. These diseases are the immunodeficiency syndrome, ataxia-telangiectasia, and the Wiskott-Aldrich syndrome. The same observation occurs among patients who have undergone an organ transplant and who receive long-term antirejection treatments and among patients suffering from acquired immunodeficiency syndrome (AIDS).

Hodgkin's lymphoma affects as many men as it does women, particularly young adults aged fifteen to thirty-five and adults aged fifty and over. The causes of the disease are unknown. Among children, lymphomas account for 10 percent of all cancers and they affect mainly adolescents aged fifteen to eighteen. The symptoms and treatments are similar to those used for adults.

Symptoms of Lymphomas

Generally, the symptoms are the same for both types of lymphomas. Patients usually consult a doctor after detecting painless lumps in the neck, armpit, or groin; in fact, these lumps are lymph nodes whose size has increased because of the lymphoma. General symptoms are excessive sweating at night, an unexplained loss of weight, fatigue, and excessive itchiness.

All organs can be affected by the lymphoma, but some, such as the spleen, the bone marrow, and the liver, are more commonly affected. Lymphomas weaken the mechanisms that fight infections; patients have a greater propensity for opportunistic infections (fungal infections, pneumocystis carinii pneumonia, and others) and must be monitored closely by doctors.

Diagnosis

When the doctor suspects that a patient is suffering from a form of lymphoma, he or she proceeds with a biopsy of a node whose size has increased. The sample is studied in a pathology laboratory and, a few hours later, the diagnosis is made.

At this point, the doctor must attempt to determine how the disease has spread (clinical phase). In other words, the doctor must determine which parts of the body have been affected.

Several diagnostic examinations are required: blood samples, a bone marrow puncture and biopsy, a radiology examination (ultrasonography, radiography, lymphography, axial tomography, etc.), and nuclear medicine examinations. Sometimes an exploratory laparotomy (abdominal surgery to evaluate whether lymph nodes and other organs are affected) is also needed.

Often demanding of the patient, these examinations are extremely important since the choice of treatment depends largely on the precision of the disease's diagnosis.

Treatment and Prognosis

Since non-Hodgkin lymphoma and Hodgkin's lymphoma do not have the same reaction to chemotherapies, we will study their treatments separately.

Hodgkin's Lymphoma

Twenty-five years ago, the survival rate for people suffering from Hodgkin's lymphoma was only 25 percent. Today, more than 90 percent of patients can be cured.

This remarkable improvement in the cure rate is the result of the discovery of new radiotherapy and chemotherapy treatment programs and new treatments involving bone marrow transplants.

Strategies Leading to a Cure First, it is necessary to establish the clinical phase of the disease; in other words, to determine to what extent it has spread to other regions and organs in the body. The doctor is careful to note the presence of symptoms such as loss of weight, fever, or excessive sweating, since the treatment that will be administered depends in part on these factors.

Hodgkin's lymphoma can be treated with simple radiotherapy when it has not spread to several regions of the body; therefore, when its clinical phase is not advanced. On the other hand, when it has spread to several regions where nodes are present (advanced clinical phase) or when the patient presents the above-mentioned symptoms, the medical team will opt for chemotherapy.

The table below outlines the treatment and the prognosis in cases of Hodgkin's lymphoma, based on the determination made at diagnosis as to how the disease has spread. The table is an overview of the treatment of Hodgkin's lymphoma; note that in oncology, each case is always considered individually by the treatment team, which, for a number of reasons, may modify a treatment program to ensure that the patient has maximum chances of survival.

Additional facts about treatment:

- In general, radiotherapy and chemotherapy are not used in combination; over the long term, doing so increases the risk of secondary leukemia.
- Regardless of the clinical phase, if there are masses of significant size, local radiotherapy may be administered, followed by chemotherapy.
- Some cases can be treated, with comparable results, by radiotherapy or chemotherapy; in particular, cases diagnosed as being in Phase II or III.
- A laparotomy is often needed in cases in Phase I or II where physical symptoms are present; if the abdominal area is affected, a chemotherapy-based treatment program may be required instead of radiotherapy.
- The chemotherapy treatment programs used to treat Hodgkin's lymphoma involve a combination of drugs. There are several combinations; the most commonly used are the MOPP (mustargene, vincristine, procarbamazine, and prednisone) combination and the ABVD (adriamycine, bleomycine, vinblastine, dtic) combination.
- The disease's progression during treatment or an early recurrence requires a change in the chemotherapy program.
- The autograft bone marrow transplant is used to treat patients who "relapse"; it is successful in 50 percent of cases.

Non-Hodgkin Lymphoma

The microscopic study of cancerous cells makes it possible to distinguish three categories of non-Hodgkin lymphoma, classified according to the potential for cell malignancy. Treatment of non-Hodgkin

Clinical Phase of Hodgkin's Lymphoma and the Resulting Treatment and Prognosis

Stage of the disease and   *Treatment*
prognosis of survival
to 5 years (%)

Phase I—only one lymph node region affected

No symptoms*   Radiotherapy
85 to 90% recovery

With symptoms   Radiotherapy or chemotherapy
75 to 80% recovery   (depending on the case)

Phase II—two or more lymph node regions, located on the same side of the diaphragm (muscle that separates the abdomen from the thorax)

No symptoms   Radiotherapy
85 to 90% recovery

With symptoms   Radiotherapy or chemotherapy
75 to 80% recovery   (depending on the case)

Phase III—two or more lymph node regions, located on both sides of the diaphragm

No symptoms   Radiotherapy or chemotherapy
70 to 80% recovery   (depending on the case)

With symptoms   Chemotherapy
60 to 70% recovery

Phase IV—one or extra-lymphatic organs affected (spleen, liver, bone marrow) with or without lymph node involvement

60% recovery   Chemotherapy

The symptoms are loss of more than 10% of total weight, fever, and excessive sweating.

lymphoma depends in large part on the category of the lymphoma in question.

Low-grade lymphomas Not very aggressive, these lymphomas are cancers that progress slowly and that involve a life expectancy of eight to twelve years. Low-grade lymphomas are incurable; it is not necessary to treat patients suffering from low-grade lymphomas with strong chemotherapies, since their considerable side effects decrease the chances of survival for such patients. A simple chemotherapy program in the form of tablets makes it possible for most patients to achieve remission. Unfortunately, recurrences are common.

Classification of Non-Hodgkin Lymphoma

Category	Potential malignancy
Low-grade lymphoma	Low level of malignancy
Intermediate lymphoma	Moderate level of malignancy
High-grade lymphoma	High level of malignancy

Intermediate lymphomas For intermediate lymphomas whose potential for malignancy is moderate, the treatment and prognosis are generally identical to those established for high-grade lymphomas.

In the experimental stage, interferon seems to be a promising treatment for intermediate lymphomas.

High-grade lymphomas These very aggressive lymphomas tend to quickly invade the lymph node and other extra-lymphatic organs such as the liver, spleen, bone marrow, lungs, digestive tract, and central nervous system. They sometimes form enormous masses that compress blood vessels, nerves, and adjacent organs, which will lead the medical team to proceed with emergency surgery to free the organs in jeopardy. The surgery will be followed by chemotherapy.

Unlike low-grade lymphomas, these lymphomas are curable when treated using various high-dose chemotherapy programs. Among the programs involving a combination of chemotherapies, the most common are MACOP-B, ProMACE-MOPP, m-BACOD, and CHOP-B; these chemotherapies are administered intravenously.

Radiotherapy is used to break down the large masses that can compress the organs adjacent to the lymphomas.

For certain high-grade lymphomas, such as Burkitt's lymphoma, surgery is needed to decrease the number of cancerous masses. Generally, such surgery is performed before chemotherapy is administered.

Autologous bone marrow transplants are used among patients who experience a recurrence after chemotherapy. Bone marrow transplant with a donor is used if the patient's bone marrow shows the presence of cancerous cells.

Prognosis Patients with low-grade lymphoma can survive for up to twelve years, but these lymphomas are incurable; over the years, these patients tend to relapse frequently and to resist chemotherapy.

Among patients with intermediate or high-grade lymphomas, the number of deaths is higher early in the disease because a number of complications arise at the outset of treatment; patients who survive beyond the critical two-year phase usually recover. The rate of survival among patients suffering from these types of lymphomas is 60 percent.

Autologous bone marrow transplants make it possible to save close to half of the patients who experience a recurrence.

In the following graph, we compare the rates of survival of patients suffering from low-grade lymphomas and those suffering from intermediate and high-grade lymphomas.

Survival of Non-Hodgkin Lymphoma

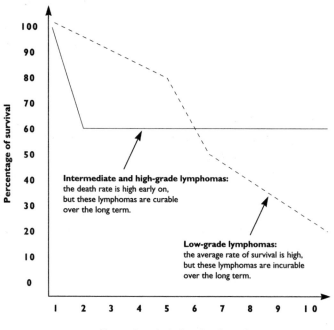

Intermediate and high-grade lymphomas: the death rate is high early on, but these lymphomas are curable over the long term.

Low-grade lymphomas: the average rate of survival is high, but these lymphomas are incurable over the long term.

Years of survival after the disease's onset

Myelomas
See Color Plate No. 13.

Myeloma is a cancer that affects a certain type of white cells known as plasma cells. These cells belong to the lymphocyte family and their main role is the manufacture of antibodies.

Myeloma accounts for 10 percent of all cancers treated in hematology.

The average age of patients suffering from the disease is sixty, but it can occur in young adults as well. Myeloma is slightly more common in men than women and it occurs at approximately the same frequency in all races.

144

Symptoms of the Disease

Myeloma often begins with vague symptoms, such as fatigue and back pain, that persist for several months, eventually leading the patient to consult a doctor.

Cancerous plasma cells multiply and invade the bones, thus causing bone pain and a decrease in the production of red cells (anemia), which results in fatigue, shortness of breath, and headaches.

This disease also causes a demineralization of the bones, called osteoporosis. Bones affected by osteoporosis lose their strength and become more sensitive to impacts, which results in frequent fractures. The most common fractures are collapsed vertebrae, which cause back pain and sometimes compresses nerves, causing sciatica and paralysis. Rib fractures cause chest pain, which can be worsened by coughing or taking deep breaths.

Myeloma also can lead to a major loss of the calcium in bones. In such instances, the calcium is released into the blood in high concentrations, which affects the proper functioning of several organs, such as the brain, muscles, and the intestines. When the calcium level in the blood is abnormally high, patients feel very weak and drowsy, are constantly thirsty, and suffer from severe nausea and vomiting.

The respiratory system is frequently affected (sinusitis and pneumonia).

Cancerous cells manufacture very large quantities of antibodies, but these are of poor quality and incomplete; consequently, they cannot protect the body against infections. These defective antibodies generally are eliminated by the kidneys. However, if they are present in too high a quantity, they can cause a phenomenon that can be compared to a river jammed with ice floes; in other words, they can accumulate in the kidneys and block filtration, causing renal failure, which is a serious complication that leads to the accumulation of water and toxic wastes in the body.

More rarely, the myeloma will form a tumor, which may compress a nerve and cause pain and paralysis in a region of the body.

The Symptoms of Myeloma

When bones are affected	Bone pain
	Bone fragility causing fractures
	Increase in the calcium level in the blood (nausea, vomiting, thirst, fatigue, confusion)
When nerves are compressed	Nerves affected by myeloma or by collapsed osteoporotic vertebrae, causing pain and paralysis in certain regions of the body, most often in the back and ribs
When the bone marrow is affected	Decrease in the production of red cells (anemia, fatigue, shortness of breath, headaches)
	Decrease in platelets (increase in bleeding)
	Decrease in white cells (respiratory system infections)
	Renal failure (fatigue, swelling in the legs, shortness of breath, protein in the urine, decrease in the quantity of urine)
When defective antibodies increase	Interference with healthy white cells decrease the immune system (increase in respiratory system infections)
	Interference with red cells (increase in the sedimentation of red cells) when the kidneys are affected.

Diagnosis

Blood samples show a major increase in abnormal antibodies (protein electrophoresis), whose monitoring is useful in following the disease's progression. The level of calcium is higher and the cell count reveals anemia and a tendency for the red cells to stick to one another and to quickly form a precipitate (increase in the rate of sedimentation).

The bone marrow puncture and biopsy show an invasion of cancerous plasma cells.

X-rays are crucial to help the doctor determine the degree to which bones have been affected; if there is a loss of bone density due to the loss of calcium in the bones (osteoporosis), the bones will be more fragile and will fracture easily. A skull X-ray can sometimes show bony lesions characteristic of myeloma.

Treatment and Prognosis

As we have just seen, myeloma is a disease that can affect several organs; consequently, treatment often requires the consultation of several specialists such as nephrologists (kidney diseases), neurologists (diseases of the nervous system), orthopedists (problems related to bones), and neurosurgeons (surgeries of the nervous system).

Improvement in the treatment of complications due to myeloma (support treatment) and the discovery of new chemotherapy treatment programs have resulted in a higher rate of survival—less than one year in the 1960s compared to more than five years in 1993. Many patients live more than ten years, and some who have undergone a bone marrow transplant experience a total remission of the disease.

Support Treatment

The first step in treatment consists of decreasing pain and reestablishing the proper functioning of any organs that have been affected.

* Bone pain: Initially, the pain will be relieved using analgesic drugs (codeine or derivatives of morphine) since it takes several days for the patient to feel the results of radiotherapy and chemotherapy; subsequently, analgesics will be administered in smaller doses.
* Nerve compression: This can be the result of the collapse of two osteoporotic vertebrae or by the myeloma itself; it is found most often in the lumbar area. When nerves are affected, emergency treatment is always required. Doctors will use radiotherapy, chemotherapy, high doses of cortisone, and sometimes even neurosurgery to

decompress the nerve as quickly as possible and to avoid serious consequences such as paralysis of a part of the body.

- Renal failure: This serious complication due to myeloma causes no pain, but seriously jeopardizes the patient's health. When it occurs rapidly (acute renal failure), doctors will ensure that a good level of hydration is maintained and will normalize the urine output using intravenous solutes and diuretics (lasix). If they cannot maintain the proper functioning of the kidneys using these methods, they will begin hemodialysis.

   Renal failure can also occur after several years (chronic renal failure) of the disease; doctors will prescribe diuretics in tablet form and the patient will be warned to avoid all situations (dehydration, the injection of iodine-based intravenous dyes) or medications that may cause kidney damage.

- Increase in the calcium level: To reestablish and maintain a proper calcium level, doctors will use drugs (cortisone, calcitonin, mithramycine) until such time as the chemotherapy has slowed down the release of calcium from the bones.

- Anemia and infections will be treated with periodic transfusions of red cells and with antibiotics administered at the first signs of infection.

Chemotherapy-based Treatment

There are several chemotherapy programs to treat patients suffering from myeloma.

In general, the first step is a program using one of two chemotherapies: melphalan or cyclophosphamide combined with prednisone. These chemotherapies can be administered in tablet form or intravenously; to prevent an increase in uric acid, another drug will also be used (allopurinol). Subsequently, interferon will be used. Thanks to these treatments, most patients experience a remission, which can last from two years to more than ten years.

The doctor will see the patient periodically and blood samples will be used to monitor abnormal antibodies since they are a good indication of how the disease is progressing. During remission, these antibodies decrease significantly in number; however, if there is a recurrence, they increase several months before the patient begins to show symptoms, which makes it possible for the doctor to modify the treatment before complications arise.

In the case of a recurrence, the doctor will use a combination of various tablet-form chemotherapies or stronger intravenous chemotherapies (carmustin, doxorubicine, vincristine). Note that some programs will make immediate use of intravenous chemotherapies.

Promising Treatments

Preliminary studies have shown that bone marrow transplants among patients with a compatible donor can lead to long-term remissions; although fragmentary, results are encouraging since they lead us to believe that it will be possible to cure myeloma.

Congenital Diseases of the Blood System

The congenital diseases we will look at are rare diseases that are present when the child is born. These diseases can significantly alter the child's state of health and can endanger his or her life if not treated rapidly. The principal congenital diseases affecting the blood are:

1. Congenital diseases of the blood cells:
   - major thalassemia
   - sickle-cell anemia
   - diseases of enzymatic insufficiency
   - aplasic anemia and Fanconi's anemia
   - congenital hypoplasia

2. Diseases of accumulation of lipids and saccharides:
   • Gaucher's disease, Niemann-Pick disease, and Hurler's disease

3. Congenital diseases of the immune system:
   • combined severe immunodeficiency
   • Wiskott-Aldrich disease
   • infantile agranulocytosis or Kostmann's disease

4. Congenital bone diseases:
   • osteopetrosis

5. Congenital diseases affecting coagulation

Congenital Diseases of the Blood Cells

Major Thalassemia and Sickle-cell Anemia
See Color Plate No. 14.

These diseases of the red blood cells exist in varying degrees of gravity, ranging from benign anemia (minor thalassemia and trace sickle-cell anemia), which causes no symptoms, to very severe forms that jeopardize the lives of young patients (major thalassemia and sickle-cell anemia).

Thalassemia and sickle-cell anemia are more common among Black individuals of African origin and among Caucasian populations in the Mediterranean region.

In these congenital diseases, a defective gene makes it impossible for red blood cells to manufacture normal hemoglobin, which is essential for the transportation of oxygen.

Symptoms of the Disease
Major thalassemia and sickle-cell anemia are very serious congenital diseases that affect young children only a few months old. These children

suffer from slow growth, anemia (pallor, fatigue, shortness of breath), and repetitive infections (otitis, bronchitis, and pneumonia). During the physical examination, the doctor will detect jaundice and discover that the liver and the spleen are enlarged. Bones may be deformed and more fragile than normal.

In the case of sickle-cell anemia, the red blood cells sometimes change shape and block the small blood vessels, which causes pain in the abdomen, thorax, bones, hands, and feet. This phenomenon is known as "vaso-occlusive crisis" and requires emergency hospitalization.

A microscopic examination of the blood reveals the presence of cells that are pale red and have lost their normal round shape. Sickle-cell anemia gets its name from the shape of the red blood cells, which resemble sickles.

The doctor will make a diagnosis based on a blood test, using electrophoresis to detect the presence of abnormal hemoglobin.

Treatment

There is no real curative treatment for these severe forms of anemia. A bone marrow transplant with a compatible donor has proven to be effective for a few young patients in whom the diseases are particularly violent.

Within a few years, gene therapy could become the treatment of choice, because it makes it possible to incorporate normal genes into the stem cells that compose the red blood cells of these young patients. These genes would provide red blood cells with a recipe to manufacture normal hemoglobin and, thus, the children would be cured for life (see "Gene Therapy" in Chapter 5).

Diseases of Enzymatic Insufficiency

Red blood cells contain enzymes, including one called glycolysis. This enzyme has a very specific role to play in maintaining the functions and the shapes of red blood cells.

The absence of glycolysis makes red blood cells more fragile. This phenomenon, in which red blood cells break apart more easily, is called hemolysis. A rare congenital defect of the glycolysis enzyme causes massive hemolysis of the red blood cells.

Symptoms of the Disease
Children who suffer from such diseases will also suffer from hemolytic-type anemia, which causes pallor, jaundice, fatigue, and shortness of breath. Often, the spleen is enlarged.

Treatment
Treatment is administered in the form of transfusions of red blood cells. Removing the spleen seems to be beneficial for some patients, and a bone marrow transplant with a compatible donor can sometimes be practiced in the most severe cases.

Aplasic Anemia and Fanconi's Anemia
Aplasic anemia and Fanconi's anemia are characterized by a progressive decrease in the formation of blood cells (red cells, white cells, and platelets) by the bone marrow.

Symptoms of the Disease
These diseases rarely involve symptoms before the age of three. The first to appear are bruising and bleeding from the gums when brushing the teeth, which are caused by the decrease in the number of platelets.

The disease progresses slowly. Since white cells decrease, the child becomes more prone to infections of the respiratory system (sinusitis, bronchitis, pneumonia); the decrease in red cells causes anemia (pallor, fatigue, headaches, and shortness of breath).

Fanconi's anemia can be present with congenital abnormalities of other parts of the body, such as an increase in skin pigmentation (large, pale brown spots), certain bone abnormalities (absence of thumbs, abnormalities in the arms, legs, and pelvis), or other abnormalities affecting the kidneys, central nervous system, heart, and gonads.

Treatment and Prognosis

The treatment of choice for young patients is a bone marrow transplant with a compatible donor, which leads to a long-term cure in more than 40 percent of cases. Other treatments make it possible to control the disease's progression, for example treatment with cortisone, androgens, and antilymphocytic globulins.

The average survival of patients who have not undergone a bone marrow transplant ranges from two to five years. The major complications are bleeding and infections. The disease sometimes progresses toward leukemia.

Congenital Hypoplasia

This form of anemia affects children at approximately two months of age. For reasons that are unknown, their bone marrow is unable to manufacture red cells. These children suffer from pallor and weakness, and these symptoms worsen progressively.

Children suffering from this disease require many blood transfusions, but the only long-term treatment is a bone marrow transplant with a compatible donor.

Diseases of Accumulation of Lipids and Saccharides

Lipids are fats and saccharides are sugars; both are found in the blood. In a child in good health, the body quickly uses absorbed fats and sugars as a source of energy. In a child suffering from a disease of accumulation, fats and sugars cannot be used properly; they accumulate in the brain, liver, spleen, and bone marrow.

These diseases are caused by an abnormality of a single gene in cells known as macrophages. Usually, macrophages eliminate toxic wastes and surplus fats and saccharides. The abnormal gene causes the accumulation of these products in the macrophages: the latter swell considerably, which hinders both their elimination of wastes and the work done by adjacent cells in the affected organ. In the bone marrow, they prevent the normal multiplication of stem cells; they also increase the size of the liver and the spleen by decreasing the levels at which they function, but the most harmful damage is to the brain, since brain cells (neurons) are unable to multiply and are particularly sensitive to compression by the macrophages.

Diseases of accumulation of lipids and saccharides are rare and found more frequently within certain ethnic groups:

- Gaucher's disease is more common among the Jewish population.
- Niemann-Pick disease is more common among the Jewish population and certain Canadians living in Nova Scotia.
- Hurler's disease is not more common in any one race.

Symptoms of the Diseases

Diseases of accumulation can progress very rapidly. Damage to the brain generally is irreversible and occurs in the first few months of life. When these diseases progress more slowly, their clinical manifestations appear over a period of a few years.

When the brain is affected: Children with these diseases are normal at birth, but after a few months, their growth slows and they present learning difficulties. Sometimes, children have episodes of convulsions, rigidity, and are prone to respiratory difficulties and problems with motor skills.

When the liver and the spleen are affected: Both organs are clogged with fats and sugars. Liver malfunction causes jaundice and coagulation problems (bruising). During a physical examination, the doctor will notice that these organs are significantly larger than normal.

When bones are affected: These diseases often affect the bone marrow. Clogging of the bone marrow prevents the normal multiplication of stem cells, which leads to a decrease in red cells and, as a result, to anemia (fatigue, pallor, and shortness of breath), a decrease in platelets (bleeding, bruising), and a decrease in white cells and, consequently, a higher risk of infections (otitis, bronchitis, pneumonia).

Bones become more fragile and fractures are not uncommon among these young children.

Genetic abnormalities: In some instances, abnormalities of the bones, heart, and urinary system will be present simultaneously.

Treatment and Prognosis

Treatment of these diseases consists of submitting the child to a very strict regimen. Unfortunately, in the most severe cases, serious effects on the brain and major complications, such as repetitive infections and hemorrhages, can lead to the death of children within the first two years of life.

A bone marrow transplant with a compatible donor is an effective form of treatment and ensures a cure for more than 50 percent of these children and, in some cases, even leads to the repair of certain types of brain damage.

Studies currently under way indicate that it may be possible to insert the missing gene; this new form of treatment, called gene therapy, could lead to very promising results.

Congenital Diseases of the Immune System

Combined Severe Immunodeficiency

Fortunately, this very serious disease is extremely rare, although it affects children in the first weeks of life.

Children are born with an immune system that does not manufacture the essential ADA enzyme (adenosine deaminase). When the immune system lacks ADA, it cannot fight any germs whatsoever. Until very recently, children suffering from this disease were forced to live in a totally aseptic environment, sheltered from infections. The smallest germ could cause their deaths.

Recently, American researchers successfully introduced a normal gene (coding the manufacture of ADA) in the immune systems of these children. This revolutionary form of treatment is called gene therapy. It enables these children to live completely normal lives.

Wiskott-Aldrich Disease

In this rare congenital disease, children suffer from skin problems (eczema) and various infections that can sometimes be serious, notably infections of the sinuses, bronchi, lungs, intestines, and occasionally, the meninges—infections caused by immunodeficiency. Since the bone marrow does not produce platelets, patients also suffer from various types of bleeding.

A bone marrow transplant with a compatible donor is the treatment of choice for these young patients.

Infantile Agranulocytosis or Kostmann's Disease

This rare congenital disease affects very young children. It is characterized by a decrease in the white cells that belong to the granulocytic family, which leads to several repetitive infections of the sinuses (sinusitis), bronchi (bronchitis), lungs (pneumonia), and at times, the blood (septicemia).

Treatment involves the use of antibiotics and close monitoring for signs of infection; cell colony stimulation factors (fsc-gm) (see "Immunotherapy" in Chapter 5) results in an increase in the number of white cells. A bone marrow transplant with a compatible donor can be effective among children who are severely affected by the decrease in white cells.

Congenital Bone Diseases

Osteopetrosis

A very severe congenital disease, osteopetrosis is characterized by the formation of extremely dense bone in the space usually occupied by bone marrow. As a result, blood cell production (red and white cells, and platelets) decreases.

Symptoms of the Disease

Children are affected by this disease from birth. The first symptoms to appear are linked to the expansion of the skull bones, whose thickness increases rapidly. This compresses the optical and auditory nerves and results in blindness and deafness. The vertebral canal also may be obstructed, which causes hydrocephalus.

Because the bone marrow gradually decreases its production of red cells, platelets, and white cells, anemia, bleeding, bruising, and infections are common and frequent.

Although very dense, the bones are extremely fragile and fractures are frequent.

Treatment and Prognosis

A bone marrow transplant with a compatible donor makes it possible to cure these children. However, the transplant must be done as soon as possible since the lesions suffered by the nervous system (nerve compression and hydrocephalus) cause irreversible damage. Without a transplant, these young patients can survive for only a few years.

Congenital Diseases Affecting Coagulation

Many congenital diseases can modify the formation of blood clots. As we saw in Chapter 2, the formation of a blood clot that will fill a break and stop a hemorrhage requires that a series of factors be set in motion.

As a result of a congenital deficiency, some of the factors shown on the following chart may be completely absent or present only in very small quantities, which slows the formation of blood clots.

The most common deficiency is Factor VIII deficiency, known as Type A hemophilia, a hereditary disease transmitted by the X chromosome and, consequently, found mainly in boys. Note that only one normal X chromosome is needed to manufacture Factor VIII, so girls usually are not affected by this disease. However, females are carriers of the disease and they transmit it to their sons in 50 percent of cases.

Children with this disease will suffer from various types of bleeding. Other types of deficiencies in coagulation factors, such as deficiencies in the Von Willebrand factor and the Factor IX deficiency, present symptoms similar to those of Type A hemophilia.

How Type A Hemophilia Is Transmitted

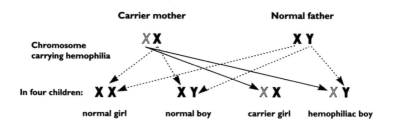

Symptoms of Hemophilia

The frequency of bleeding among hemophiliacs varies from one boy to another, depending on whether Factor VIII is totally or partially absent. Thus, some boys will suffer from hemorrhages at a very early age, while in others, the disease will be discovered only after several years, for example, during a dental surgery procedure where the child's bleeding is abnormal.

The most common bleeding occurs in the large joints (hemarthrosis), such as the knees, shoulders, and hips. In the long term, repetitive hemorrhages such as these can lead to joint deformities. Blood can also accumulate in the muscles (hematoma), which causes pain and stiffness, and painless bleeding may occur in the digestive tract (stomach).

The first sign of hemophilia may be abundant and persistent bleeding after minor surgery, such as a tooth extraction or a tonsillectomy.

Diagnosis is made using blood tests designed to evaluate the reaction times of the various stages of coagulation and by analyzing individual coagulation factors.

Treatment and Prognosis

In the past, most children suffering from hemophilia and other congenital diseases affecting coagulation died of uncontrollable hemorrhaging. Today, the deficient factors are replaced by coagulation factors taken from the blood of normal subjects. These factors are administered intravenously at regular intervals and enable patients to life lives that are almost completely normal.

To avoid the risk of hemorrhage, however, violent sports and some dangerous physical activities are proscribed.

A multidisciplinary team including hematologists and orthopedists ensures that constant monitoring and blood tests will be used to evaluate coagulation and the condition of joints.

The Treatment of Blood Diseases

Only fifteen years ago, malignant blood diseases such as leukemia, lymphoma, or aplasia left little hope for survival. Today, for many patients the recovery rate is over 70 percent. In large part, this success is linked to the joint use of several forms of treatment, namely chemotherapy, radiotherapy, bone marrow transplants, surgery, and new medical technologies such as immunotherapy and gene therapy. Take for example chronic myelogenous leukemia: In 1980, this disease killed 80 percent of patients after two years. Today, bone marrow transplants lead to recovery in more than 70 percent of patients.

Treatments have only one goal: curing the patient while causing minimal side effects so that the best possible quality of life can be maintained. These diseases and their treatment are often extremely difficult, both physically and psychologically, for both patients and their families; therefore, it is crucial that all involved have a good understanding of the healing and recovery process and that each participates actively in that process.

Personal research into relaxation techniques—such as acupuncture, massage therapy, meditation, visualization—should be considered; such techniques counter stress and make it easier to weather the situation.

Alternative medicines are not discussed in this publication, but people who would like more details on such approaches should consult the Suggested Reading list at the end of the book.

Medical Strategies
Leading to Recovery

The time when doctors treated several different types of cancers with only one weapon, two or three chemotherapy agents, is long gone. Today, an ultraspecialized form of medicine, called oncology, helps us to combat these serious diseases.

In oncology, each drug that is used is first the object of comparative studies and statistics proving its effectiveness and superiority over another therapeutic agent.

The treatment and recovery of patients suffering from a malignant blood disease calls for the concerted action of several medical and paramedical workers.

The treatment of each patient involves a number of specific steps that must be taken one by one, at the appropriate time:

1. Establishing a *precise diagnosis* of the disease. A precise diagnosis is arrived at through microscopic, biochemical, cytogenetic, and immunological studies. Precision is crucial in the choice of a treatment program.
2. Evaluating the degree to which the disease has spread (*clinical stage*). This step also plays a role in the choice of a treatment program. Thus, in the case of Hodgkin's lymphoma, chemotherapy is sometimes combined with radiotherapy; on the other hand, in the case of leukemias that have spread extensively into the central nervous system, a sample of cerebrospinal fluid showing the presence of cancerous cells will lead to additional radiotherapy treatment.

To adequately determine the clinical stage, the doctor will

proceed with an in-depth physical examination and will prescribe laboratory and diagnostic tests that can be highly sophisticated at times, such as computer-assisted radiology, ultrasonography, and nuclear medicine.

3. Choosing the *appropriate treatment program*. In the treatment of a given cancer, several types of anticancer drugs are used in combination and administered in very precise doses, at very precise intervals; this is what doctors refer to as a treatment program. In short, programs are recipes combining several ingredients (chemotherapies) to ensure the best rate of recovery while causing the fewest possible side effects.

These programs are designated by abbreviations composed of the initials of each of the drugs used. For example, CHOP is a program often used in the treatment of non-Hodgkin lymphomas (cancer of the lymph nodes), and is composed of cyclophosphamide, adriamycine (in this instance, exceptionally, the "H" does not correspond to the first letter of the word), oncovin, and prednisone. Patients who have a CHOP treatment come to the oncology outpatient clinic every three weeks, over a period of twenty-four weeks. Cyclophosphamide, adriamycine, and oncovin are administered intravenously, while prednisone is ingested in tablet form over the following five days.

Radiotherapy is sometimes combined with chemotherapy; for example, for children suffering from acute lymphocytic leukemia, irradiation of the central nervous system is part of several treatment programs.

There are a great many chemotherapy treatment programs, and as new discoveries improve recovery rates and decrease the number of side effects, they undergo constant change.

4. The treatment itself, which includes five sequences: *induction, prophylaxis of certain organs, consolidation, maintenance, and support.*
   a) The *induction treatment.* The objective of this first sequence is to destroy as quickly as possible the highest number of leukemic cells while ensuring the survival of stem cells in the bone marrow and

the proper functioning of other vital organs. Essentially, induction aims to achieve remission; in other words, the disappearance of the clinical and microscopic signs of the disease.

During an induction treatment, the patient is hospitalized for a period of several weeks, and doctors administer combinations of three or four chemotherapeutic agents during this period.

b) The prophylactic treatment of certain organs. Some patients have a strong propensity to show a recurrence of the disease in certain organs. To prevent such recurrences, a treatment described as prophylactic or a specific prevention treatment is administered to these organs as soon as the induction treatment ends. Before prophylactic treatment of the central nervous system among patients suffering from acute lymphocytic leukemia was used, recurrences in this part of the body accounted for 50 to 60 percent of all recurrences. The radio-therapy-based prophylactic treatment makes it possible to decrease significantly (to less than 20 percent) the number of recurrences in the central nervous system and to increase the rate of recovery.

c) The consolidation (intensification) treatment. This treatment begins immediately after the induction treatment.

Consolidation makes it possible to destroy the leukemic cells that may have survived the induction treatment and it is particularly effective among patients suffering from leukemias whose prognosis is poor.

d) The maintenance treatment. Depending on the case, maintenance treatment begins immediately after the induction or consolidation treatment. Maintenance treatment usually includes sequences of several types of chemotherapy at regular intervals of two or three weeks, over a period of twenty-four to thirty-six months. The maintenance treatment prevents recurrences over the long term.

e) The support treatment. This sequence is designed to prevent and cure the complications resulting from the disease or its treatment. There are many potential complications: infections, hemorrhaging, anemia, kidney, liver or lung disease, loss of weight, an imbalance in electrolyte elements (potassium, sodium, calcium, phosphorus, and magnesium) in the blood, and an increase in wastes generated by cancerous cells or their treatment (uric acid). Thus, throughout the treatment, several blood samples will be taken to monitor the proper functioning of all of the body's organs.

5. Resumption of treatment in case of recurrence. If there is a recurrence, the medical team will undertake a second induction treatment, different from the first, and will consider the possibility of a bone marrow transplant. Sometimes, depending on the sickness, a bone marrow transplant will be done after the induction treatment.

Chemotherapy

Chemotherapy was first used in the 1950s. It is based on the principle of differential toxicity: the substances used are toxic for all living cells, but they are even more toxic for dividing cells, notably cancerous cells.

Over the years, numerous chemotherapy agents have been synthesized; in this section we will examine their action mechanisms and their main side effects.

Chemotherapy Defined

In this form of treatment, the doctor uses several types of drugs that stop the division of cancerous cells. These drugs, described as anticancer or antineoplastic drugs, can be administered intravenously, orally in the form of capsules or tablets, or directly into the cerebrospinal fluid to treat or prevent the infiltration of leukemic cells into the central nervous system.

The Action Mechanisms of Chemotherapy

Anticancer agents act by stopping the cells that are dividing rapidly. The agents penetrate the cell and attack the nucleus by intervening in the usual functioning of the DNA chain or by blocking certain chemical reactions within the cell. The cells are then unable to complete their division and, eventually, they die.

However, cancerous cells that are not dividing when the chemotherapy is administered are not killed. To counter this problem, doctors sometimes use anticancer agents that act at different times and on distinct parts of the cell. The doctor also may prescribe a maintenance treatment that makes it possible to destroy cancerous cells described as "dormant" or "sleeping"; in other words, cancerous cells that do not divide for long periods of time. These cells awaken after several months, and it is at this point that maintenance treatment is vital.

Despite these complex treatments, not all cancerous cells are destroyed. Some are naturally resistant to induction treatment, while over time others become insensitive to chemotherapy and can cause a recurrence. This phenomenon is known as cancerous resistance.

Cancerous Resistance

Cancerous cells become resistant to chemotherapy by various means, including the manufacture of a substance (p-glycoprotein) that pumps drugs out from the cells, thus preventing chemotherapeutic agents from penetrating the cell.

Several researchers are working to find a solution to cancerous resistance. Thus, recent discoveries have shown that drugs and antibodies directed against p-glycoprotein are able to neutralize its effect completely. The solution to the problem of cancerous resistance may be the manufacture of large quantities of these antibodies.

For the moment, to destroy resistant cells doctors use treatment programs that include drugs that are more powerful or different from the initial drugs used to treat the patient.

Side Effects of Chemotherapy

In the human body, many cells divide very rapidly without being cancerous. Stem cells in the bone marrow, cells on the surface of the intestines, cells that form sperm and ovules, and follicles at the base of hairs all multiply rapidly.

As mentioned previously, chemotherapy agents penetrate cancerous cells, but they also penetrate healthy cells, thus inhibiting their growth.

The secondary effects caused by chemotherapy can appear immediately or a few weeks after treatment.

Important Points about Side Effects
- Most side effects are reversible.
- Side effects vary from one patient to another and from one treatment to another.
- Some side effects lessen over the course of the treatment.
- It is important to be familiar with side effects to recognize their symptoms quickly and to counter the anxiety linked to treatment.
- Some reactions can occur very quickly, in "acute" form, while others occur only a few days or a few weeks later, in "delayed" form. Nausea and vomiting are "acute" secondary effects that occur a few minutes or a few hours after the administration of chemotherapy, while hair loss is a "delayed" reaction, occurring several days after treatment begins.

Main Side Effects
1. Effects on the bone marrow. A few days after the administration of chemotherapy, there is a decrease in the manufacture of blood cells; this is known as the suppression of "the medullary function" or "hematopoiesis function."

   If the number of red cells is low, the patient will develop anemia;

a decrease in the number of platelets will increase the possibility of hemorrhaging; and a decrease in the number of white cells will increase the risk of infection.

To prevent such complications, the doctor must sometimes decrease the chemotherapy dosage.

2. Effects on the digestive tract. The digestive tract, which runs from the mouth to the anus, is composed of cells that are sensitive to certain chemotherapies.

In the mouth, there may be ulcerations, inflammation of the gums, and insensitivity to the taste of foods.

Irritations extend to the esophagus and the stomach, which leads to difficulty swallowing, heartburn, nausea, and vomiting.

Anxiety leads to a significant increase in the symptoms of nausea and vomiting. It is not uncommon to encounter patients who experience nausea at the mere sight of the chemotherapy room. Studies conducted among consenting patients have shown that placebos (drugs administered in the same way as chemotherapy drugs, but containing only water and sugar) can cause nausea and vomiting among very anxious patients. It has also been shown that administering chemotherapy at night, while the patient is sleeping, decreases symptoms significantly. It is very important that the patient find ways to relax and control stress and anxiety.

3. Effects on the reproductive system. Anticancer treatments can cause infertility in both men and women.

Effects on the male reproductive system. In the testicles, thousands of cells known as spermatogonia cells divide throughout the patient's lifetime to form sperm. Spermatogonia cells are very sensitive to chemotherapies and radiation. Therefore, their growth can be totally and irreversibly inhibited as a result of intensive treatment.

In the case of pubescent male patients, some sperm can be frozen and preserved for several years.

Effects on the female reproductive system. Side effects on the female reproductive system are more common among young women. During adolescence, cells within the ovaries (ovocytes) multiply intensely. After a few divisions, the ovocytes become ovules. When a young woman reaches the age of eighteen, ovule formation ceases; the maximum number of ovules has been produced. Subsequently, one of these ovules will be released during each menstrual cycle, until menopause.

Ovocytes are very sensitive to anticancer treatments. Thus, among young female adolescents receiving chemotherapy, the risk of sterility is higher than among adult females.

Unfortunately, it is difficult to remove and conserve ovules, but new techniques such as in vitro fertilization may make it possible to counter infertility among young women suffering from cancer.

Menstrual cycles are often disturbed: they begin early or they slow down, they are intermittent or they stop completely. If bleeding is too heavy, menstruation must be stopped using replacement hormones.

Neither men nor women show any decrease in libido directly linked to chemotherapy; it is usually a temporary side effect.

4. Loss of hair (alopecia). Hair loss may occur after some types of chemotherapy.

Alopecia occurs gradually, a few weeks after the treatment begins, but is reversible in most cases. Hair on legs, the pubis, the chest, and the abdomen usually does not fall out because it grows very slowly and, therefore, is not very sensitive to chemotherapy. The beard tends to fall out during treatment, but it grows normally when treatment ends. Note that baldness can progress further after chemotherapy.

New hair grows at the rate of approximately 0.04 to 0.08 inches (0.5 mm) per day. It is usually finer and tends to curl.

Some people also lose their finger- and toenails, but the nails usually grow back following treatment.

5. Effects on the skin. Certain drugs can cause redness and itchiness; others, such as myleran, tend to increase the skin's pigmentation. The skin becomes more sensitive to the sun; therefore, patients should avoid long periods of exposure.

The Future of Chemotherapy: Homing Drugs

Homing drugs are molecules that have the property of traveling specifically to cancerous cells while ignoring the healthy cells in our organism. Therefore, their effectiveness is increased and they have fewer side effects.

Two types of homing drugs are now the focus of intense research: drugs attached to antibodies and drugs incorporated into microspheres (liposomes or polymers).

Drugs Attached to Antibodies
On the surface of their membrane, some cancerous cells have antigens that are specific to them. It is possible to attach chemotherapy molecules to antibodies that are complementary to these antigens. The antibody-chemotherapy complexes then attach only to cancerous cells carrying antigens. When they arrive at their destination, the cancerous cells absorb the chemotherapy molecules and the latter disrupt internal systems and prevent cell division.

The drugs attached to the antibodies present two major problems for researchers. First, not all cancerous cells have distinct antigens on the surface of their membrane; consequently, several types of cancer cannot be treated using this method. Second, on average at least one thousand chemotherapy molecules are required to destroy a single cancerous cell; however, no more than one hundred molecules can be sent at any one time using this technique.

Microspheres (Liposomes or Polymers)
Microspheres are synthetic particles ten to fifty times smaller than red

cells. Hundreds of thousands of chemotherapy molecules are incorporated into them when they are manufactured.

Injected into the blood, loaded with their chemotherapy agents, microspheres travel to cancerous cells, which absorb them; as a result, high numbers of chemotherapy molecules are released directly into the cancerous cells. Microspheres make it possible to bring a large quantity of chemotherapy agents to the inside of cancerous cells.

However, this technique involves a major problem for researchers: cancerous cells are not the only type of cells that absorb microspheres. In fact, white cells, stem cells in the bone marrow, and macrophages located in the liver all absorb them as well, and these cells are particularly sensitive to chemotherapy. Therefore, the use of microspheres is limited when the immune system, blood cells, and liver have been affected.

To circumvent the problems posed by homing drugs, scientists are attempting to attach antibodies to microspheres, since antibodies make it possible to direct the microspheres solely toward cancerous cells. With a considerable loading capacity, microspheres can ensure that an adequate amount of chemotherapy agents is carried to the inside of cancerous cells.

The combination of these two homing drugs makes it possible to circumvent the specificity of cancerous cells and the minimal dose required to stop their multiplication. During preliminary studies, these drugs have proven to be very effective for several types of cancers.

Radiotherapy

Radiotherapy is a form of treatment that uses invisible rays, such as gamma rays, X-rays, and electrons. These high-energy rays attack the nuclei of cells undergoing division. By breaking the DNA chain located in the nuclei, the rays disrupt the cancerous cells and stop their growth.

Unfortunately, radiotherapy is not specific to cancerous cells; thus, some organs of the human body, such as the bone marrow, the scalp, the intestines, and the reproductive organs, are particularly sensitive to these rays.

Diseases Treated by Radiotherapy

Radiotherapy is used to treat patients suffering from advanced Hodgkin's lymphomas. It is also used to shrink large tumors sometimes found in lymphomas and myelomas involving a compression of the spinal cord or the nerves.

The treatment of lymphocytic leukemia requires the use of radiotherapy in combination with chemotherapy. Among children, for example, it is used on the skull and the spinal column to destroy the leukemic cells that may have penetrated the central nervous system.

During a bone marrow transplant, radiotherapy is sometimes applied to the entire body; this technique is known as total body irradiation.

Method of Treatment

Radiotherapy requires that the tumor's location be determined extremely precisely. This calls for sophisticated methods such as computer-assisted axial tomography, commonly referred to as scanography; ultrasonography; nuclear medicine; and magnetic resonance. When the tumor has been located, markings are applied to the skin and used as indicators delimiting the treatment site.

It is also necessary to calibrate very precisely the dose of radiation applied to a given area. The dose is expressed in RADS (a unit of radiation dose absorbed by a cancerous tumor or an organ).

Radiotherapy equipment consists of a gamma ray generator operating on cobalt 60, a betatron, and a linear accelerator that produce electrons or high-energy X-rays.

Given the emission of radiation, the equipment is installed in rooms insulated with thick lead walls and, usually, the radiotherapy department is located in a remote part of the hospital, either in the basement or in an adjacent building. The equipment is large in size and pivots so that the rays can be concentrated on the tumor site.

Depending on the type of cancer and its location, the radiotherapist will decide on the number of sessions and on the total dose of radiation (number of RADS) to be administered.

Side Effects

Side effects appear after a certain number of sessions: the skin around the irradiated site becomes red and the patient may experience fatigue, loss of appetite, nausea, vomiting, and diarrhea.

These side effects cause patients to feel anxiety, nervousness, and often, exhaustion. Discuss your problems with the treatment team; they can help you find ways to better tolerate these unpleasant effects (see Chapter 6).

Surgery

As we saw in Chapter 3, surgery plays an important part in establishing the diagnosis of certain blood diseases. For example, when exploring lymph node diseases such as lymphoma, it is crucial to proceed with biopsies of the node to arrive at an accurate diagnosis.

However, doctors make very little use of surgery for curative purposes in the treatment of these diseases, since they tend to infiltrate several organs rapidly and at the same time, which makes surgery impossible.

In the case of some blood diseases, surgery is used jointly with chemotherapies and radiotherapy with the objective of a curative treatment. In the case of Burkitt's lymphoma, before the patient receives chemotherapy treatment, the surgeon removes the largest cancerous masses. In the case of certain rare leukemias, such as hairy cell leukemia, doctors sometimes remove the spleen (splenectomy).

Surgery is indispensable when certain cancerous nodes compress vital organs. In such instances, the surgeon removes the nodes to relieve the organs in question, which makes a chemotherapy treatment program possible.

The surgeon also intervenes to install various intravenous catheters, which remain in place for several weeks. These catheters make it possible to administer drugs, to perform transfusions, and to take blood samples without the need for repeated and unpleasant "needles" in the patient's arm.

Bone Marrow Transplant

Bone marrow transplant can cure several malignant blood diseases; its therapeutic success has given it a place of choice in oncology around the world.

From the purely human standpoint, bone marrow transplant is a unique treatment, calling several emotions into play. From the medical standpoint, it is complex, grouping several scientific concepts and therapeutic methods into a single treatment.

The medical team is composed of doctors with specialized training in bone marrow transplants, either through research or clinically.

The nursing team is skilled in all transplant techniques and the specialized care required by transplant recipients.

The dietetic department calculates the nutritional needs of each patient and develops menus that can satisfy them while complying with the aseptic standards that apply to the patient's room.

Pharmacists monitor the drug doses that are absorbed by the patient's body to ensure compliance with therapeutic measures.

The social services team offers material support to the patient and the family.

Finally, several individuals work in the shadows; for example, members of the cleaning staff, laboratory technicians, all of whom work in close cooperation with doctors and nurses.

History of the Bone Marrow Transplant

The first bone marrow transplants were done in France. In the 1960s, the victims of a nuclear power station accident in Yugoslavia were transported to the Curie Institute. Since radiation had destroyed their bone marrow, these patients could no longer manufacture the blood cells required for their survival. Despite only rudimentary knowledge of the compatibility between donors and recipients, doctors went ahead with transplants nonetheless. Most recipients died as the result of numerous severe complications, such as rejection, hemorrhaging, and infections, but a few patients survived the mortal consequences of the nuclear accident. The bone marrow transplant was born.

A little over thirty-five years later, more than forty thousand individuals have undergone this form of treatment.

Bone marrow transplant has become the treatment of choice for several malignant blood diseases, such as leukemias, lymphomas, aplasias, and some congenital diseases. A new type of transplant, known as the autologous transplant, makes it possible to cure patients without using an "external donor." This procedure increases the bone marrow transplant's potential to cure patients.

In the thirty-five-odd years of transplants, many beautiful stories of recovery have been recorded, some of them miraculous. The two following accounts are a good illustration of the promise held by the bone marrow transplant.

The "Ping-Pong" Transplant: Bone Marrow Traveling from One Generation to Another

Emsworth, a fishing village in England. In 1980, Stuart, aged ten, contracted a form of leukemia whose severe prognosis left him only a few weeks to live. Unfortunately, HLA (human leucocyte antigen) compatibility tests failed to identify a perfectly compatible donor; only Alan, Stuart's father, had a few HLAs in common with his son.

Doctors were reluctant to try a transplant; the risk of acute rejection was considerable and could lead to death, just as Stuart's leukemia could. However, they decided to go ahead with the transplant; the operation was an unqualified success and Stuart recovered.

Seven years later, returning from a fishing expedition on the high seas, Alan complained of bone pain and bruising on his legs. A visit to the family doctor quickly led to the diagnosis of a fatal disease: by a very unfortunate coincidence, Alan was now suffering from leukemia.

Alan needed a bone marrow transplant, but none of his brothers or sisters was compatible. The doctors turned to the only person likely to be in a position to donate marrow: Alan's son, Stuart. And so Alan received his own marrow, which he had given to his son a few years earlier.

Today, both father and son have recovered.

"The most touching aspect of this story was seeing Stuart's emotion as his gave his marrow to his father—the same marrow he had received from Alan seven years previously," commented one of the treatment team's doctors, Dr. Powles.

Scientists dubbed the transfer of marrow between father and son "the ping-pong transplant."

Bone Marrow Traveling from One Country to Another

Quebec, Canada, 1989. Celine, suffering from an incurable disease, was saved by a bone marrow transplant. Her donor, found in a registry of American donors, was a man who lived near Washington, D.C. David was a perfectly compatible donor who lived many hundreds of miles from Celine.

Although the donor's name is usually confidential, a few months after the transplant Celine and David met. Charged with emotion, the meeting was an occasion for warm embraces and tears.

David described his feelings: "My mother used to say that blood was the most precious of all liquids, and that my sister was the most precious person I could ever have in my life. Now, my blood is Celine's blood. I have a second sister in my life, so I decided to visit her."

Today, hundreds of patients are saved thanks to volunteer donor registries.

To facilitate comprehension of bone marrow transplant, we will answer a series of questions that are frequently put to doctors.

1. What Is the Difference Between Bone Marrow and the Fluid Surrounding the Spinal Cord?

Many people confuse bone marrow with the fluid surrounding the spinal cord.

As seen previously, bone marrow is formed of stem cells that multiply nonstop to manufacture platelets, white and red cells. It is particularly abundant in the pelvis and sternum.

The spinal cord is an extension of the brain. It is composed of nerve fibers that run down the center of the spinal column and extend between the vertebrae to form nerves. A lesion in the spinal cord will lead to paralysis of the entire part of the body located below the lesion. For example, a lesion may occur when the spinal column is fractured. Since nerve fibers do not have the ability to regenerate themselves, spinal cord fluid cannot be transplanted using current techniques.

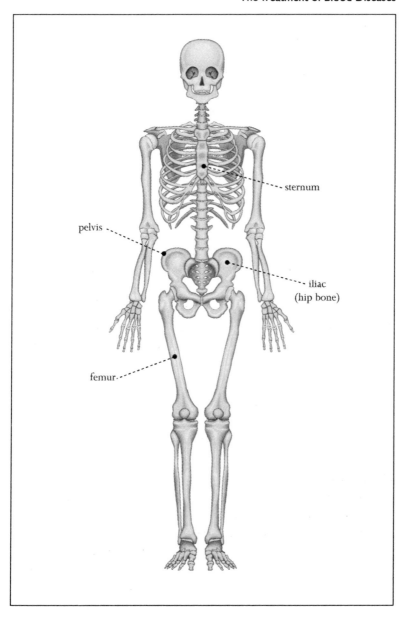

**The pelvis and the sternum are sites
where bone marrow is rich in stem cells**

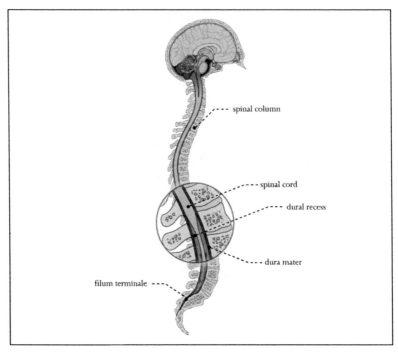

The spinal cord and the nerves are extentions of the brain

2. What Diseases Can Be Treated with a Bone Marrow Transplant?

The diseases we will discuss here are malignant; patients suffering from these diseases have a life expectancy of only a few months. Before deciding on a bone marrow transplant, the medical team will evaluate all other treatment possibilities. Other non-neoplastic diseases affecting bone marrow cells or their progeny can also be treated by bone marrow transplantation.

The decision to proceed with a bone marrow transplant is based on the evaluation of the patient and several specific aspects related to the patient's overall health. Thus, the presence of diseases affecting the

Diseases That Can Be Treated with a Bone Marrow Transplant

Diseases in adults	Particularities of the diseases	Survival rate (3 years)
Chronic myelogenous leukemia	This leukemia tends to be very stable during the first year (chronic phase); subsequently, it becomes very aggressive (high-grade phase and blastic phase). The bone marrow transplant must be done when the patient is in the chronic phase, since the survival rate is significantly higher in this phase. Generally, doctors wait one year before doing a transplant on a patient in the chronic phase. Among patients in the high-grade or blastic phase, the transplant is done within a shorter period of time because recurrences are common. The type of transplant used is the donor transplant; for the moment, the autologous transplant is in the research stage.	65–75% (chronic phase) 40% (high-grade phase) 15% (blastic phase)
Acute myeloblastic leukemia	Patients undergo a transplant after the first remission, since recurrences are rapid and severe. The autologous transplant with selective depletion of cancerous cells can also be used when no donor is available.	50–60% (donor transplant) 40–45% (autologous transplant)
Acute lymphoblastic leukemia	In most cases, the donor transplant is done after the first remission. The autologous transplant with selective depletion of cancerous cells is possible.	50–60% (donor transplant) 35–40% (autologous transplant)
Aplastic anemia	The donor transplant must be done rapidly because the short-term complications associated with aplasia are very severe.	60–70%
Myeloma	The donor transplant is possible among patients aged less than 55 whose general state of health permits it.	50% (preliminary results)
Pre-leukemias (myelodysplasic syndrome)	The donor bone marrow transplant gives excellent results; the autologous transplant is not possible for the moment.	60%
Lymphoma	The transplant makes it possible to cure patients suffering from lymphomas who experience a recurrence after conventional treatments. The autologous transplant is the main type of transplant used to treat these patients; donor transplants may be used in some instances.	45–50%
Solid tumors	Bone marrow transplant is currently under study for several types of cancer such as cancer of the breast, lungs, or testicles, or melanoma. Preliminary results are encouraging; generally, all tumors disappear.	

N.B.: The survival rates and certain particularities of the bone marrow transplant presented in this table are subject to constant change due to the continuous introduction of new and more effective treatment programs.

heart, lungs, and liver and severe infections can delay or even elimi-nate the transplant procedure.

Age is an important factor; with some exceptions, candidates must be at least fifty-five years old.

Individuals suffering from AIDS cannot be treated with a bone marrow transplant since the virus is not eliminated by chemotherapy; therefore, it survives in the body, quickly reinfecting newly trans-planted white cells and stem cells.

Before proceeding with a bone marrow transplant, the cancerous disease must be in remission. This remission is achieved through chemotherapy and radiotherapy. When the clinical and microscopic signs of the disease disappear, doctors can go ahead with the trans-plant procedure.

3. What Are the Different Types of Bone Marrow Transplant?

There are two types of bone marrow transplant: the allogenic bone marrow transplant, which involves a donor, and the autologous bone marrow transplant, in which the patient serves as his or her own donor.

The Allogenic Bone Marrow Transplant

The "allo" prefix means "of different origin." Therefore, this transplant uses bone marrow from another person (donor). The donor can be a member of the patient's family; in this instance we refer to a "related allograft."

If the donor has been found in a volunteer donor registry, we refer to an "unrelated allograft."

The Autologous Transplant

The autologous bone marrow transplant, is one in which the patient serves as his or her own donor.

The bone marrow is removed and frozen; it can be kept for several weeks, even years, before being retransfused into the patient.

4. Why Is a Bone Marrow Transplant Used to Treat a Patient?

All of the cancerous diseases discussed in this book can be controlled for a certain time using basic treatments: chemotherapies and radiotherapy.

The major problem is that, eventually, cancerous cells become resistant to these treatments and are no longer destroyed by the usual chemotherapy doses. Doctors therefore must administer increasingly stronger doses of chemotherapy and radiotherapy. However, the stem cells in the bone marrow are very sensitive to these treatments. If the chemotherapy dose goes beyond a certain level, they will also be destroyed. Consequently, doctors are limited in the way in which they use chemotherapy and radiotherapy.

However, the transplant generates new bone marrow after intense chemotherapy treatment. This "healthy" marrow takes over and, within a few weeks, produces completely normal blood. The bone marrow transplant thus makes it possible to give very strong doses of chemotherapy while maintaining the blood's biological functions.

5. What Determines the Compatibility Between a Donor and a Recipient?

On the surface of all of the cells in our body there are small structures known as HLAs (human leucocyte antigens). HLAs are specific to each individual; they could even be described as each individual's "natural social insurance number."

White cells recognize any foreign cell that does not have HLAs identical to their own. This is called the rejection reaction.

HLAs are divided into four groups: A, B, C, and D. The A, B, and D groups are the most important for compatibility.

There are several HLA subtypes (see the table of HLAs identified in humans, page 183); thus, in the Type A HLA group, there are forty-nine different subtypes; in the Type B HLA group, there are twenty-four; in the Type C HLA group, there are eleven; and in the Types D and DR HLA groups, there are forty-six.

In the general population, some of these subtypes are more common than others. Note that Type DR HLA determines the outcome of a compatibility known as the mixed lymphocytic culture.

Each individual has two HLA groups that are not identical. Thus, an HLA mapping can look like this:

Robert Patenaude's HLA

A1—A3
B8—B7
Cw1—Cw8
Dw9—Dw26

As you can see, the number of possible HLA permutations is huge; thus, within the general population, the chance of finding two individuals with the same HLAs varies from 1 in 8,000 to 1 in 500,000.

HLAs are transmitted genetically. Half of them come from the mother, and the other half come from the father. It is easier to find a compatible donor among brothers and sisters who belong to the same family, since parents transmit only half of their HLAs to each of the children. The probability of compatibility is 25 percent or one chance in four for each member of the family. The gender of the donor and the recipient are of very little importance for a bone marrow transplant. In rare instances, one of the parents can act as a donor for his or her child.

HLA Groups and Blood Groups
It is important to point out that HLA groups are completely different

HLAs Identified in Humans*

A	B	C	D	DR
A1	B5	Cw1	Dw1	DR1
A2	B7	Cw2	Dw2	DR2
A3	B8	Cw3	Dw3	DR3
A9	B12	Cw4	Dw4	DR4
A10	B13	Cw5	Dw5	DR5
A11	B14	Cw6	Dw6	DRw6
Aw19	B15	Cw7	Dw7	DR7
A23(9)	B16	Cw8	Dw8	DRw8
A24(9)	B17	Cw9(w3)	Dw9	DR9
A25(10)	B18	Cw10(w3)	Dw10(w7)	DRw10
A26(10)	B21	Cw11	Dw11(w7)	DRw11(5)
A28	Bw22		Dw12	DRw12(5)
A29(w19)	B27		Dw13	DRw13(w6)
A30(w19)	B35		Dw14	DRw14(w6)
A31(w19)	B37		Dw15	Drw14(w6)
A32(w19)	B38(16)		Dw16	DRw15(2)
Aw33(w19)	B39(16)		Dw17(w7)	DRw16(2)
Aw34(10)	B40		Dw18(w6)	DRw17(3)
Aw36	Bw41		Dw19(w6)	DRw18(3)
Aw43	Bw42		Dw20	
Aw66(10)	B44(12)		Dw21	DRw52
Aw68(28)	B45(12)		Dw22	
Aw69(28)	Bw46		Dw23	DRw53
Aw74(w19)	Bw47		Dw24	
	Bw48		Dw25	
	B49(21)		Dw26	
	Bw50(21)			
	B51(5)			
	Bw52(5)			
	Bw53			
	Bw54(w22)			
	Bw55(w22)			
	Bw56(w22)			
	Bw57(17)			
	Bw58(17)			
	Bw59			
	Bw60(40)			
	Bw61(40)			
	Bw63(15)			
	Bw64(14)			
	Bw65(14)			
	Bw67			
	Bw70			
	Bw71(w70)			
	Bw72(w70)			
	Bw73			
	Bw75(15)			
	Bw76(15)			
	B77(15)			
	Bw4			
	Bw6			

* The small "w" after the HLAs signifies "work," since researchers are working on these HLAs to better define them.

Source: Provided by Bodmer, W.F. et al. (1987), "Nomenclature of factors of the HLA system," in Dupont, B. (editor). Immunology of HLA, Vol. I. (New York: Springer-Verlag, 1989).

from the blood groups we hear of frequently (for example, the A, B, and O groups).

A difference in blood groups between donors and recipients is not a contraindication to a transplant, since after a few weeks, the graft will produce new blood that will belong to the donor's group.

A difference in blood groups simply calls for different preparation in the days preceding the transplant. The doctor will proceed with a plasma exchange in the recipient; this technique makes it possible to remove the antibodies and prevent a transfusional reaction during the transplant, since the graft has the same blood group as the blood it manufactures.

When the new cells appear, the patient's blood group will be identical to the donor's (for example, my blood type was O before my transplant, and now, seventeen years later, I belong to the B blood group, the same as my donor, my sister Diane).

6. Who Can Be a Bone Marrow Donor?

As seen previously, donors usually come from the patient's family, in which case we refer to a "related transplant." If the donor comes from outside the family, we refer to an "unrelated transplant."

The chances of finding a compatible donor in the general population are very small. For example, the chance of your neighbor being compatible with you range from 1 in 8,000 to 1 in 500,000.

Bone Marrow Donor Registries

Throughout the world, there are several bone marrow donor registries or banks. Donor banks are simply computerized lists containing the names and addresses of individuals who have agreed to submit to blood tests to determine their HLA group. Only a few cubic centimeters of blood is needed to determine the HLA group, and the procedure takes only a few minutes. Subsequently, the individual's name and

HLA group are entered in the computer list and the individual becomes part of the bone marrow donor bank.

Internationally, there are several donor registries; it is estimated that there are more than five million registered donors worldwide. (On the Web, see http://bmdw.leidenuniv.ml/.) People who agree to be donors may one day be called upon to save a life.

The Future

We have long known that the umbilical cord and placenta are rich in stem cells capable of multiplying and reproducing bone marrow. Recently, researchers have developed a technique to recover the stem cells in the umbilical cord and placenta immediately after a baby's birth. There is no risk for the newborn's health, since the cord and placenta are usually destroyed after the birth. These stem cells are then frozen and can be kept throughout a lifetime. Their number is sufficient for them to be reused during a bone marrow transplant.

To date, a few transplants using this type of stem cells have been practiced successfully. In a few years, perhaps we will witness the creation of banks set up to freeze stem cells taken from each newborn's umbilical cord. These stem cells could be retransfused, if necessary, when the child becomes an adolescent or adult and is stricken with a malignant blood disease. To some extent, they would constitute a "biological life insurance policy."

7. What Procedures Must Be Followed to Become a Bone Marrow Donor?

If you want to donate your bone marrow, you should contact the hematology secretarial service in a hospital where bone marrow transplants are practiced. You will be given an appointment for blood tests—only a few test tubes are needed to proceed with HLA typing—and your HLA type will be included in the computerized donor list.

If You Are Lucky

If your HLA type is compatible with a person suffering from a malignant blood disease, whether that person is a brother, a sister, or an unknown person living on the other side of the world, you will experience very strong emotions—your donation may save a life.

Before proceeding with the transplant, a second series of blood samples are taken for even more specific tests to determine compatibility with the patient.

Several weeks go by between the final compatibility tests and the removal of the donated bone marrow. This time is needed for the patient's anticancer treatments.

A few weeks before the procedure, a doctor meets with the donor to do a general physical examination and to take a sample of one or two units of blood (a pint or 450 cc). To prevent weakness and to ensure proper recovery, the sample is conserved and retransfused to the donor on the same day that the donated bone marrow is removed by the multiple punctures method. (See question 8.) This transfusion is particularly important among donors who are small in stature and go to the multiple punctures method (see below).

In the case of a bone marrow donation with a unrelated donor, the names of the donor and the recipient are kept secret. However, the doctor will be pleased to inform the donor of the transplant's outcome, even if it occurs in a different country.

8. How Is Bone Marrow Removed from a Donor?

Many people think that the bone marrow transplant is a very complicated surgical procedure; however, the procedure is relatively simple.

As we have seen, bone marrow has a liquid consistency and is rich in stem cells. Capable of regenerating blood cells, stem cells are concentrated in the pelvis and sternum. Recently, researchers have discovered that stem cells are also found in the blood, in small quantities.

With injection of a new medication, granulocytic colonies stimulating factor (G-CSF), it is possible to obtain a big concentration of stem cells in the blood.

There are two methods of removing these cells: directly from the pelvic bone through *multiple punctures*, or through *apheresis*, which consists of removing the stem cells found in the blood. The apheresis method is easier and more popular.

Removal Through Apheresis

Apheresis is a technique that makes it possible to separate the blood's different cells, concentrate the stem cells, and collect them.

Twenty-four to 48 hours before the apheresis, the donor will receive a dose of granulocytic colonies stimulating factor (G-CSF). This medication is given intravenously in one dose.

The technique requires the installation of two intravenous catheters, one in each arm. Through one of the catheters, blood is sent to a centrifuge that separates the cells. The stem cells are removed and collected in a sterilized plastic bag. The blood that is emptied of stem cells is returned to the donor through the second catheter.

Each apheresis session lasts approximately two hours. One or two apheresis sessions are required to obtain a sufficient number of stem cells for the transplant. The stem cells are sent to the patient's room to be transfused. In case of an autologous transplant, the marrow is sent to the laboratory to be treated and frozen. There is no retransfusion of donor's blood in the apheresis method.

The advantage of this technique is that it is danger-free and does not require general anesthesia in an operating room setting.

Removal Through Multiple Punctures

The donor will be hospitalized the day before the operation and will be reexamined before the operation. In the operating room, the donor or the patient (in the case of an autologous transplant) is put to sleep under a general anesthetic. Certain conditions may require an epidural anesthesia.

Doctors take close to two hundred samples using very rigid needles. The total quantity of bone marrow collected is approximately one quart, and the intervention lasts approximately two hours.

The marrow is then filtered to remove bone particles and is immediately sent to the patient's room to be transfused. In the case of an autologous graft, the marrow is sent to the laboratory to be treated and frozen.

Finally, a unit of the donor's blood is retransfused after the intervention.

The donor recovers very quickly from the operation; he or she leaves the hospital the following day, and a few days after intervention is able to resume all normal activities.

9. Are There Any Risks Involved in Being a Donor?

For donors in good health who used the apheresis method, the risks are minimal, and might even be described as nonexistent. For those who used the multiple punctures method, lower back pain is the only discomfort experienced by the donor, and it quickly disappears after a little exercise.

Serious complications are very rare and they are usually due to the general anesthetic; at times, donors suffer from hemorrhaging, infections, or cardiovascular problems. These reversible complications are easily treated. To date, thousands of transplants have been done worldwide and no donor has died of complications related to a transplant.

The donor's bone marrow or stem cells regenerate in two or three weeks and the quantity taken from the donor is replaced rapidly.

The removal of the bone marrow or stem cells has no effect whatsoever on the immune system or the vital functions of the donor's blood. Therefore, the risk of complications and side effects are minute for the donor.

10. What Are the Steps in a Bone Marrow Transplant?

When all controls and compatibility tests have been completed, the patient is admitted to the hospital. At this point, the bone marrow transplant procedure has truly begun.

Stage 1

A flexible venous catheter is installed at the chest level. This intervention is done under local anesthesia in the operating room.

Stage 2

A chemotherapy-based anticancer treatment program with or without radiotherapy is begun.

This step lasts eight to twelve days and is followed by a two-day rest period to eliminate all chemotherapy agents that could hinder the bone marrow from being accepted by the body. For some patients, new chemotherapy agents could be given by pills at home and patients are admitted to hospital just two or three days before the bone marrow transplant.

Stage 3

The marrow is transfused through the venous catheter.

Through a mechanism that we do not understand at present, the stem cells reenter the tiny veins in the bones and multiply there. It takes a few weeks before they begin to manufacture new blood.

Stage 4: From the Day of the Transplant to Release from the Hospital

Since the patient is deprived of white cells for a period of four to six weeks and is consequently sensitive to infections, he or she must stay in a completely aseptic room. A sophisticated air filtration system eliminates airborne germs. Visitors wear a lab coat and a mask, and they must wash their hands thoroughly before entering the room.

The four weeks following the transplant are particularly difficult. The side effects of the chemotherapy, such as inflammation of the throat and the digestive tract, are sometimes sufficiently severe to prevent the patient from eating properly. Nutrients are replaced by intravenous feeding.

Throughout this period, the patient could receive multiple transfusions of platelets and red cells, to prevent hemorrhaging and anemia. At times, the patient's immune system becomes refractory to platelet transfusions; in other words, it begins to manufacture antibodies that destroy the transfused platelets. In such cases, the donor is called back to provide platelets, which the patient's system will accept since his or her immune system is now identical to the donor's immune system. This platelet removal technique, identical to apheresis, is known as thrombopheresis; it is danger-free and does not require the donor's hospitalization.

For several weeks, drugs will be administered to prevent rejection reactions and infections. Although these drugs are hard to absorb, they are very important in the prevention of serious complications. In the case of autologous transplants, antirejection drugs are not needed, since the patient receives his or her own marrow; therefore, rejection is impossible.

By the time the new marrow produces blood cells in adequate quantity, transplant recipients have been hospitalized for close to one month. Patients can be released as soon as their immune systems are ready.

The improvements of medical research in bone marrow transplant have reduced the average hospitalized time, from the 2 1/2 months of 10 years ago to just a month today.

Stage 5

Throughout the next six months, the patient must visit the outpatient clinic on a regular basis.

The patient must wear a mask and avoid contact with individuals who have colds, flus, or pneumonia; he or she must not take needless risks, since the immune system requires several months to return to normal.

During the fourth month, the patient undergoes a complete physical examination. If all is normal, over a period of a few weeks the doctor gradually will decrease the drugs used to prevent graft versus host (GVH) reaction and infections; eventually, they will be completely stopped. If signs of GVH reaction reappear, patients must begin taking the drugs again, gradually eliminating them several months later.

After a transplant, a new series of vaccinations is not required.

Physical examinations and laboratory tests are repeated each year over a period of five years.

11. What Are the Particularities of the Autologous Transplant?

The autologous transplant is a technique in which the patient serves as his or her own donor. Bone marrow is removed in the same way as it is for transplants with compatible donors.

After the procedure, the marrow is sent directly to a laboratory. There, it is used in one of two ways:

1. It is frozen immediately; this is usually the case if it must be used to treat lymphomas and malignant tumors (breast cancer).
2. A new laboratory technique, called "selective depletion" or "purging," is used to eliminate the majority of leukemic or lymphomatic cells in the bone marrow sample. This procedure makes it possible to "wash" the marrow that has been infiltrated by cancerous cells to keep only those stem cells that are viable and in good health. After the washing, the marrow is sent for freezing.

When the cancerous cells found in certain lymphocytic and myelogenous leukemias and in certain lymphomas have infiltrated the bone marrow, selective depletion makes it possible for patients with no compatible donor to undergo an autologous transplant. Unfortunately, not all leukemias or all lymphomas can be treated through the use of the autologous technique and selective depletion;

but here again, research is advancing quickly and at times a new treatment can be only a few months away.

Freezing techniques make it possible to conserve the marrow for several weeks, giving doctors the time they need to administer strong doses of chemotherapy to eliminate cancer cells from the patient's body.

The patient will receive his or her own marrow through transfusion and must go through the same treatment stages as patients who receive a transplant from compatible donors.

During an autologous transplant, a rejection or GVH reaction is impossible since the patient is receiving his or her own bone marrow. Therefore, no antirejection drugs are needed. The rate of infection and the average number of days of hospitalization are lower than they are in the case of allografts.

Average Number of Days of Hospitalization, Including Days Required for Chemotherapy

Transplant with donor (allograft)	30 to 45 days
Autologous transplant (autograft)	25 to 35 days

The autologous graft is a technique that leads doctors to be very hopeful with regard to the successful treatment of certain types of lymphomas and leukemias. It has been tested on other forms of cancer, such as cancer of the breast, lungs, and testicles, melanomas, and neuroblastomas. Although fragmentary, results are very encouraging, particularly in the case of breast cancer.

12. What Are the Rejection Reactions During a Bone Marrow Transplant?

During a marrow transplant, two types of rejection reactions are possible.

The HVG Reaction

When the patient rejects the donor's bone marrow, the reaction is referred to as HVG (host versus graft—the host is the patient). Fortunately, this type of rejection is very rare.

It occurs a short time after the transfusion of new marrow; at that time, a large quantity of stem cells is destroyed. Thus, new blood will take a great deal of time to form.

The GVH Reaction

The rejection reaction observed most frequently is called GVH (graft versus host). It occurs when the donor's cells reject some of the patient's organs.

The GVH reaction can occur between the second and tenth week after the transplant; it can be very strong or can manifest itself through only slight symptoms.

When the GVH reaction is intense and occurs early on, it is described as an acute GVH reaction. Thanks to certain new drugs, the acute GVH reaction has become rare.

When the GVH reaction is weak and occurs in the weeks following the transplant, it is described as a chronic GVH reaction. The chronic GVH reaction is the most common type; it affects approximately 40 percent of transplant recipients. GVH is more frequent with unrelated bone marrow transplants when the donor has been found in a volunteer donor registry.

The organs most commonly affected are the skin, tear glands, salivary glands, liver, and intestines. The symptoms of this reaction are the following:

- Skin. The apparition of painless redness, similar to a sunburn.
- Tear glands and salivary glands. At the outset, there is a short phase during which secretions increase, but glands quickly stop producing tears and saliva. Patients will complain that their mouth and eyes are dry, but not painful.

- Liver. Pain is rarely present when the liver is affected; at times, jaundice may accompany sensitivity in the region where the liver is located.
- Intestines. Diarrhea and stomach cramps are frequently linked to a GVH reaction of the intestines.

The GVH reaction is usually controlled through the use of drugs such as cyclosporin and cortisone; it tends to disappear during the first year. Nonetheless, approximately half of all patients who experience a GVH reaction must take drugs over a longer period of time.

Studies have shown that patients experiencing a GVH reaction are at less risk of experiencing a recurrence of their leukemia. It seems that the GVH reaction destroys the rare malignant cells that have survived the chemotherapy. This phenomenon is known as the GVL (graft versus leukemia) reaction. Through the GVL's action, the GVH reaction provides protection against recurrences of the leukemia.

13. What Complications Can Occur During a Bone Marrow Transplant?

Apart from rejection and the GVH reaction, complications resulting from a bone marrow transplant are infections, hemorrhaging, the side effects of chemotherapy, and recurrences.

During the period of hospitalization, the infectious complications that may occur include pneumonia, enteritis, and infections at the intravenous catheter sites. After the first four months, infections are increasingly rare. However, patients receiving antirejection drugs are sensitive to infections of the lungs and the skin, such as shingles.

Hemorrhages are rare and affect mainly the regions that experience the side effects of chemotherapy (for example, the mouth, throat, stomach, and bladder). Patients often find traces of blood in their spittle, or notice that their urine is pinkish. However, most of these forms of bleeding are temporary and benign and they are not alarming.

Chemotherapy can affect the liver, lungs, kidneys, and bladder. All of these complications usually are well controlled through medical treatments, and they rarely leave lasting effects.

14. What Are the Long-Term Side Effects of a Bone Marrow Transplant?

The strong doses of chemotherapy and radiotherapy used in treatment programs can have long-term side effects.

As a result of its effects on the reproductive system, most patients, both male and female, become sterile. Women often stop menstruating and experience early menopause. In such instances, they receive replacement hormone therapy. Among men, sperm production is interrupted, but this does not affect sexual functions per se. Before the transplant, the sperm of postpubescent patients can be frozen, should they plan to have children in the future.

Hair loss is a temporary problem; hair begins to grow back in the third week after the transplant. On the other hand, among patients who suffer from baldness before the transplant and among patients experiencing a GVH reaction, hair can grow back very slowly.

The skin has a "tanned" tint for several years. It also may remain sensitive for a long time following an infection such as shingles (herpes zoster skin infection).

The eyes can present cataracts, especially among patients who have received radiotherapy and cortisone.

Patients who experience a GVH reaction, and who must take drugs such as cyclosporin and cortisone as a result, can experience increased pilosity, weight gain, and roundness of the face. If the GVH treatment continues over several years, cyclosporin may cause high blood pressure and cortisone may cause diabetes and osteoporosis. These effects disappear quickly when drug doses are decreased.

In rare cases, the side effects caused by chemotherapy treatments can lead to serious after effects. For example, obliterating bronchiolitis and pulmonary fibrosis can affect the patient's respiratory functions, and kidneys may be affected by renal failure.

The donor's allergies are often transmitted to the transplant recipient. Thus, a donor suffering from seasonal rhinitis (hay fever or an allergy to ragweed) can transmit the allergy to the transplant recipient.

All of these side effects can be worrisome, but to handle them effectively, the patient should become familiar with them. And it is important to know that the bone marrow transplant is a technique that is in constant development. The complications mentioned here were discovered in the course of studies conducted over the past twenty years. In that period, treatment programs have changed considerably and some of these complications have become extremely rare. Other programs aimed at minimizing side effects while treating cancerous cells more effectively are currently under study.

15. What Are the Specifics of Bone Marrow Transplants among Children?

Bone marrow transplants practiced on children involve approximately the same procedures, techniques, and compatible donor selection as those practiced on adults.

However, there are some differences in indications, complications, and the psychological effects of the disease and the treatment on the young patient and his or her family.

Is Age a Limiting Factor?
Absolutely not. In one case, a baby of two and a half months received a bone marrow transplant.

Furthermore, in the case of a disease of accumulation of saccharides or lipids, for example, where the brain can be affected and mental retardation, deafness, or blindness can result, it is imperative to proceed with a transplant as soon as possible, since such complications are irreversible (see "Congenital Diseases of the Blood System" in Chapter 4).

Donors must be sufficiently big in stature to provide an adequate quantity of marrow; the quantity is calculated based on the recipient's size, since an insufficient quantity could cause serious problems for the patient. Recently doctors have developed a technique to perform bone marrow transplants from stem cells recovered from the umbilical cord.

Note that in certain countries, for a minor donor, a judge's authorization is required before proceeding with removal of a bone marrow sample. This procedure is simplified through the involvement of social services professionals or an attorney.

Indications of Transplants among Children

Contrary to what occurs with adults, where transplants are practiced after the first remission, in most cases involving children, doctors wait until there is a recurrence of the leukemia before proceeding with a transplant. The reason is that more than 60 percent of children will be cured through conventional treatment based on chemotherapy and radiotherapy of the central nervous system. This rate is comparable to the rate obtained through bone marrow transplants; therefore, there is no advantage to an immediate transplant.

For cases of very aggressive leukemia and in cases of recurrence, the transplant offers additional hope of recovery.

For certain types of very aggressive leukemia, the medical team will opt for a bone marrow transplant after the first remission.

Generally, patients who require a transplant are the same types of patients found among adults: those suffering from aplastic anemia, lymphomas, acute leukemias, chronic leukemias and certain congenital diseases, such as diseases of accumulation of lipids and saccharides, disorders of the red cells (Fanconi's anemia, thalassemia, etc.), osteopetrosis, and immunodeficiencies.

Complications

Note that there are a few differences compared to what occurs among adults:

- In general, children tolerate chemotherapy better than adults do.
- The GVH reaction and pulmonary complications (pneumonia, bronchitis, fibrosis) are less common among children.
- There is often a slowdown in growth, which means that these children are slightly shorter than average when they become adults.
- High doses of chemotherapy result in sterility among both girls and boys. However, when chemotherapy treatments involving lower doses are used, as is the case with aplastic anemia, the reproductive system is often unaffected.
- When the transplant is practiced on prepubescent girls, their reproductive systems are often unaffected. In addition, a study conducted among young girls who received a transplant and who bore children showed that their children are in excellent health and suffer from no long-term after effects.
- Girls often suffer from ovarian hormone deficiency, which manifests itself through a stoppage in the menstrual cycle or through irregular cycles. To counter this problem, the doctor will prescribe replacement hormones.
- If boys are postpubescent, their sperm can be frozen for later use. The sperm can be conserved throughout the patient's lifetime. While the reproductive system is affected by anticancer treatments, sexual functions per se are unaffected.

The Psychological Effect

Throughout the transplant period, and even after the young patient has returned home, particular attention should be paid to the psychological effect the lengthy illness has on the child and other members of the family.

In addition to undergoing the stress of the disease and its treatment, the sick child is forced to remain in an aseptic room for several weeks and he or she does not always understand the reasons behind therapeutic interventions.

Some children react aggressively, regress, or withdraw into total silence.

Diseases in Children that Can Be Treated through a Bone Marrow Transplant

In the case of cancerous blood diseases (leukemias and lymphomas), there must be a remission of the disease, achieved through chemotherapy and radiotherapy, before doctors proceed with a transplant.

Diseases in children	Particularities
Acute lymphoblastic leukemia	For most young patients suffering from lymphoblastic leukemias, the bone marrow transplant is used only if the leukemia recurs, namely after a second remission.
	This decision is based on the fact that conventional chemotherapy and radiotherapy treatments cure young patients in approximately 60 percent of all cases.
	The transplant is considered as a second possibility for patients who experience a recurrence; in such cases, the recovery rate is approximately 35 to 50 percent for transplants with a donor and 30 to 40 percent for autologous transplants.
	For young patients suffering from very high-risk leukemias, the medical team can proceed with a transplant immediately after the first remission.
Acute myeloblastic leukemia	For this type of leukemia, there are two therapeutic strategies. The first consists of using a transplant with a donor as soon as remission is achieved; the recovery rate is approximately 60 percent in this instance. The second consists of proceeding with a transplant only if there is a recurrence of the leukemia (which occurs among approximately 40 to 50 percent of young patients after a first remission); at this point, the recovery rate drops to 40 percent. The choice of treatment is made following a consultation involving the doctors on the medical team. For the moment, the autologous transplant is rarely used, since recurrences are common.
Acute myeloblastic leukemia	This leukemia accounts for less than 1 percent of leukemias found in children under eighteen. The transplant is practiced during the first year, since the leukemia tends to be stable (chronic phase) at the onset of the disease. Subsequently (high-grade phase or blastic phase), it becomes difficult to treat.

199

Diseases in children	Particularities
Chronic myelogenous leukemia	The results of the transplant with a donor are excellent: 50 to 70 percent of recipients are cured if the transplant is practiced when the leukemia is in the chronic phase; the recovery rate drops to 40 percent if the leukemia is in the high-grade phase and to 30 percent if it is in the blastic phase. The autologous transplant is still only an experimental technique.
Lymphoma	The transplant makes it possible to cure 60 percent of young patients suffering from lymphomas who experience a recurrence after a conventional chemotherapy or radiotherapy treatment, or both. The autologous transplant is mainly used to treat these patients; sometimes, a transplant with a donor is used.
Aplastic anemia	A transplant with a donor must be practiced quickly, since complications from aplastic anemia are very severe; the rate of success is 70 percent.
Congenital diseases	Several diseases are transmitted genetically from one generation to the next. These diseases jeopardize the survival of young children who contract them. The bone marrow transplant (with a donor) constitutes their sole chance of recovery.

These diseases include accumulation of saccharides and lipids, osteopetrosis, severe immunodeficiencies, and diseases of the red cells (major thalassemia, Fanconi's anemia). The recovery rate is 45 to 50 percent for most patients. |
| Solid tumors | The bone marrow transplant is currently in the experimental stage for several types of cancer among children: neuroblastoma, osteocarcinoma, melanoma, and tumors of the testicle and breast. Preliminary results are encouraging: in general, tumors disappear, but recurrences are common. Researchers are working on improving treatment programs that lead to the elimination of a high number of cancerous cells and a reduction in the recurrence rate. |

N.B.: The survival rates and certain particularities of the bone marrow transplant presented in this table are subject to constant change due to the continuous introduction of new and more effective treatment programs.

The sick child requires much more attention from his or her parents, which leads to anxiety in brother and sisters, who sometimes feel abandoned. And throughout these difficulties, parents must also carry out their day-to-day duties, which go on despite the tragedy of illness. It is crucial that the treatment team provide as much assistance as possible, while respecting the family's intimacy and the personality and reaction of each individual.

The Future

Since families now have fewer children (only 30 percent of children have a compatible family donor), research is now focused on autologous transplants with cancerous cell depletion and control of the GVH reaction in unrelated bone marrow transplant.

The number of unrelated donor lists is increasing steadily; thanks to computerization and communications technologies, doctors now have access to banks of five million donors living on the other side of the world.

The future offers much hope and science is progressing consistently as techniques improve. One day, leukemia and other cancers will be a thing of the past.

Immunotherapy

Immunology is a new science that studies the functioning of our defense mechanisms. The immune system, or defense system, is composed of thousands of cells that form a powerful army capable of protecting us against infections and other aggressions from our environment.

Throughout our lives, the defense system reacts constantly against viruses and bacteria; furthermore, it causes inflammatory reactions that are indispensable to the healing of burns or lacerations of the skin.

For the past several years, the hypothesis that our immune system plays a role in the defense against cancer has elicited a great deal of interest among researchers. The development of a cancer may be closely linked to the proper functioning of our defense system. A deficient immune system cannot recognize a cancerous cell in time; the latter is then free to multiply and form a malignant tumor. Consequently, we wonder whether a hyperefficient immune system could recognize cancerous cells and destroy them quickly, thus suppressing the cancer as soon as it appears.

Patients suffering from immunodeficiency (a weakened state of the defense system) are more sensitive to certain cancers, such as cancers of the skin and certain lymphomas. Conversely, patients whose immune systems are very energetic, such as a subject who has received a bone marrow transplant and who experiences a GVH reaction, are at less risk of a leukemic recurrence. In this graft versus leukemia reaction, new transplanted cells are capable of destroying the cancerous cells that have survived chemotherapy.

Researchers are just beginning to understand the functioning of the immune system, which is one of the most complicated and one of the least well known of the human body's systems. The immune system functions like a true army; it has billions of white cells, antibodies, and natural substances that act as messengers between our white cells.

For example, when an infection is present, the result is a fierce battle between our immune system and the aggressors. Thus, when a cold rhinovirus attacks our throat, the following sequence of events takes place:

1. White cells recognize the virus as foreign and quickly secrete particular messengers, which attract other white cells to drive back the invader. This is the first counterattack.
2. In the meantime, other cells manufacture a second type of messenger, which activates the multiplication of white cells to launch a final attack against the invader. This explains the increase in the number of white cells in the blood when an infection is present.

3. To prevent a new infection, Type B lymphocytic white cells keep the invader's portrait in memory; if needed, they will manufacture an antibody against it.

Thus, our organism will be protected for life against this virus branch. Unfortunately, since there are hundreds of different viruses, this process offers no protection against other types of infections.

The "messengers" referred to here are natural substances that researchers have discovered recently and that transmit information between cells. The mechanisms used to transmit messages between white cells coordinate and program the proper functioning of our defense system.

For the past several years, certain synthetic messengers and antibodies (monoclonal antibodies) have been used in the treatment of malignant blood diseases.

The Immune System's Messengers

The principal messengers that have clinical applications are interferon, granulocytic colonies stimulating factors, interleukin, and monoclonal antibodies.

Interferon

This messenger is manufactured by white cells (lymphocytes and macrophages). It activates the immune system to fight viral infections and even certain malignant blood diseases.

In the past few years, researchers have successful synthesized interferon in the laboratory; it can also be obtained in sufficient quantity for medical use.

Interferon is used as a treatment in three malignant blood diseases: chronic myelogenous leukemia, hairy cell leukemia, and myeloma. In these three cases, it stimulates the defense system and slows down the growth of cancerous cells. Interferon is administered daily by subcutaneous injection; the treatment is comparable to that given to a diabetic patient who requires daily injections of insulin.

Thanks to interferon, most patients experience remissions that last several years, with the need for conventional chemotherapy.

Granulocytic colonies stimulating factors (GCSF)

These natural messengers favor the multiplication of stem cells in the bone marrow and increase the number of granulocytic-type white cells in the blood.

It is well known that one of the side effects of chemotherapy is a decrease in the multiplication of cells in the bone marrow; this phenomenon is known as hematopoiesis suppression. Growth factors accelerate the resumption of the bone marrow's activity after intense chemotherapy or a bone marrow transplant. Thus, the number of granulocytic-type white cells (white cells whose role is crucial in the defense against bacterial infections) returns to a normal level more rapidly, which decreases the risk of infection and the number of days during which the patient must remain hospitalized in an aseptic room.

Studies have also shown that patients suffering from myelodysplasic syndrome and children suffering from congenital agranulocytosis can benefit from the stimulation factors found in cell colonies.

Interleukin

This substance is produced by the macrophages and by some white cells.

Interleukin includes numerous subtypes. These substances play a major role as messengers during immune reactions. They increase the multiplication of lymphocytes, stimulating the bone marrow and causing fever during infections.

From a therapeutic standpoint, they are the focus of intense research. Recently, researchers discovered that they allow the multiplication of specialized lymphocytes in the recognition and destruction of certain forms of cancer. Tests conducted by Dr. Rosenberg in cases of skin cancer (melanomas) are very promising and open the door to a new form of treatment.

Monoclonal Antibodies

These antibodies, manufactured in very large quantities, attack certain particles and even certain cells in a very specific way.

Recently, researchers succeeded in producing antibodies capable of destroying certain leukemic cells while saving health cells. This technique is used in the bone marrow transplant with selective depletion of cancerous cells.

Immunotherapy is a form of treatment that will take on more importance in the coming years. Several new messengers and monoclonal antibodies are currently under study (interleukin, the tumoral necrosis factor) and preliminary results are very promising.

Gene Therapy

In medicine, bold hypotheses sometimes arise, making it possible to bring research a giant step forward.

In 1952, in Paris, researchers Watson and Crick presented the spiraled double chain structure known as DNA, outlining its crucial role in coding and transferring vital information to all living cells. Today, all researchers recognize the fundamental role of DNA.

DNA forms a long spiraling helix located in the nucleus of each cell. The helix is divided into small sections known as genes. The genes contain a code that incites the cell to manufacture proteins, enzymes, and antibodies. The production of these substances allows the cell to accomplish the work that is specific to it. Thus, B lymphocytic-type white cells have genes used to manufacture the antibodies that defend the organism against viruses and other microorganisms. Red cells have genes that code the fabrication of a protein (hemoglobin) that catch oxygen. Hemoglobin transports oxygen to all of the body's organs.

All cells have genes that allow them to play a precise role; this is

205

called gene expression. Sometimes, the expression of a gene can be defective; the affected cells are then unable to accomplish their work and, inevitably, there are consequences for the individual's health.

Severe immunodeficiency is a congenital disease caused by a defective gene located inside the white cells. These cells can no longer secrete an enzyme called ADA (adenosine deaminase). An immune system deprived of ADA is unable to combat even the most inoffensive of germs. Until very recently, children suffering from this disease were forced to live in a totally aseptic environment. This was the case with David, a young American boy who in the 1960s was known as "the boy in the bubble." He suffered from immunodeficiency and, before dying of a fatal infection, lived for seventeen years in confinement in a sterile space.

In the past few years, researchers have succeeded in incorporating a normal gene coding the manufacture of ADA in the white cells and stem cells of children found to be immunodeficient at birth. Cells treated in this way can destroy bacteria and viruses, making it possible for these children to live completely normal lives. This revolutionary new form of treatment is known as gene therapy.

This new science studies genes; techniques are developed to isolate and transfer genes from one cell to another. Very recently, researchers found a way to recognize and isolate faulty genes (oncogene) causing certain cancers. These oncogenes are genes that have undergone mutation and whose information code has become erroneous as a result, ordering the cell to multiply nonstop, which results in the formation of a first cancerous cell.

Only forty-five years after the discovery made by Watson and Crick, we are at the dawn of a new form of treatment that will make it possible to replace defective or deleterious genes, thus curing diseases at their source. Gene therapy will probably be available in the 21st century for several diseases whose cause is a gene deregulation, such as hereditary diseases (cystic fibrosis, immunodeficiency, major thalassemia, etc.) and acquired diseases (cancers, for example). It will be possible to recognize, inhibit, and replace a gene that has become defective, or to make the immune system aggressive toward cancerous cells. Within a few years, gene therapy will surely play a major role in the treatment of malignant blood diseases.

Practical Advice for Patients ⬛ **6**

This chapter contains practical advice to help patients prevent certain side effects of chemotherapy and radiotherapy. To better understand the side effects involved in various forms of treatment, read Chapter 5.

Radiotherapy and several anticancer drugs cause nausea and vomiting. Some medications can help to reduce the intensity of such reactions, but they cannot be eliminated completely. These medications are more effective if they are administered before the anticancer treatments. To counter side effects, some treatment centers use complementary techniques, such as relaxation exercises and hypnosis.

Mouth-Related Problems

Mouth-related problems (irritation and ulceration) can be reduced through the regular use of mouthwash. However, to be effective, the mouthwash must be used after each meal.

Do not use commercial mouthwashes; they contain alcohol, which dries out the tissues of the mouth and increases the level of pain. This simple and easy recipe results in an excellent mouthwash: Dissolve one teaspoon of salt and one teaspoon of baking soda in one quart of water, at room temperature.

Use glycerin-coated swabs, absorbent cotton, and a very soft toothbrush.

Painful mouth sores can be relieved by applying a local anesthetic (xylocaine) prescribed by a doctor. This medication can be very beneficial if applied immediately before meals.

Patients should have any cavities seen to before undertaking chemotherapy.

If mouth lesions are persistent and painful, discuss them with your doctor; they can be a sign of a fungal infection (moniliasis).

Loss of Appetite and Nausea

A well-balanced diet is very important during treatments. The body needs a healthy diet to regain its strength and to repair the damage done by the disease and the treatment.

The following tips can help the patient cope with loss of appetite:

- Eat when you are hungry, even if it happens to be between meals.
- Eat often; eat small meals throughout the day.
- Keep nutritious, low-sugar foods on hand: cheese, vegetables, milk, fresh or dried fruit, and fruit juices; vary your meals.
- On days when you feel hungrier, eat more to gain weight.
- Drinking a glass of wine or beer with meals can sometimes help to stimulate the appetite.
- Some dishes are easy to prepare and offer good nutritional value: vegetable soups (cream of tomato, cream of mushroom, etc.), beef consomme, chicken bouillon, etc.
- When you feel well, prepare a few full meals for future use.

If this advice doesn't help, speak to a doctor, nurse, or dietitian about the possibility of using food supplements.

Gastrointestinal Problems

If discomfort occurs after treatments, avoid eating for several hours before each treatment; if it occurs before or during the treatment, eat only a very light meal before the treatment.

Use these tips if you have observed bowel problems or diarrhea with previous chemotherapy:

- Follow a liquid diet (soft drinks without carbonated water, no caffeine, no milk, and no alcohol; juice and sports drinks like Gatorade are good) to help your stomach and intestines work properly.
- Avoid very cold or very hot foods.
- Let carbonated drinks sit until they stop bubbling.
- When you begin to feel better, gradually add low-fiber foods to your diet: rice, bananas, fruit-flavored gelatin, applesauce, mashed potatoes, biscuits, and crackers.
- Avoid foods that can cause cramps, such as coffee, beans or peas, broccoli, cauliflower, cabbage, very spicy or high-fat food, and sweets; do not chew gum.
- Avoid drinking milk or eating dairy products if they seem to make your diarrhea worse.

Heartburn and Stomachaches

Heartburn and stomachaches caused by drugs such as cortisone usually can be reduced by taking antacids (Maalox, Sulcrate, Tagamet, Zantac, etc.).

Beware! If you vomit blood or if your stool is black, consult your doctor immediately; these problems can be the symptoms of a stomach ulcer.

Weight Gain

Cortisone has the unfortunate effect of causing water retention and weight gain. Weight gain can be partially controlled by avoiding high-fat foods and limiting your salt intake. For example, avoid salty snack foods such as chips and pretzels.

Skin and Hair

Irritation of the skin and tissue burns may occur at sites where radiotherapy is applied or where drugs such as vincristine and adriamycine are injected. The symptoms—redness, inflammation, and pain—appear a few days after the injection. Tell the doctor immediately; quick treatment can prevent severe burns and ulceration.

Avoid irritating the skin needlessly. Do not use soap, cosmetics, perfume, salves, or sunlamps. Do not expose your skin to the sun or to extreme cold.

If the skin on your face is irritated and if you have to shave, use an electric razor.

211

Hair loss may occur following the use of adriamycine, cyclophos-phamide, methotrexate, or vincristine, or when radiotherapy is applied to the skull. There is no effective means of avoiding this secondary effect, but hair loss is usually temporary; a few weeks after the treatment, hair begins to grow back.

Fatigue, Anxiety, and Emotional Problems

Many people experience fatigue during the treatment period. The human body uses a great deal of energy to fight the disease and to repair the damage caused by treatments. Patients should rest as often as possible and should plan activities to ensure that there are no obstacles to their well-being or comfort.

Insomnia and extreme anxiety are common during the treatment period. Doctors can temporarily prescribe sleeping pills for very nervous patients.

It is important for family and friends to realize that, during the treatment period, the patient's behavior will be different. Some people feel exhausted or nervous.

It is crucial to adopt a positive attitude, both intellectually and emotionally, with regard to treatments and to cancer in general. Speaking to someone you feel comfortable with—such as a doctor, nurse, technician, social services professional, chaplain, relative, or friend—can be extremely beneficial.

Some people find emotional and physical comfort in meditation and relaxation exercises. It is easy to find books on these subjects or to register for introductory courses.

Feel free to discuss your worries and questions with a doctor, nurse or technician. Make a list of the medications you use. Before taking any medication whatsoever, even aspirin, ask a doctor or a nurse for advice.

When Should You Call a Doctor?

Call a doctor in the following circumstances:

- urticaria-type allergic reactions (hives); inflammation of the hands, feet, or eyelids
- appearance of bruising or bleeding; remember that you can also detect signs of hemorrhaging in the urine (pink, red, or brown) and in stool (red or black)
- shortness of breath during the administration of daunorubicine, adriamycine, or methotrexate
- thirst or excessive urination during the administration of prednisone or dexamethasone
- blood in the urine and pain during or after the administration of cyclophosphamide
- jaundice (yellowish tint to the skin and eyes) during the administration of a drug, regardless of what it is
- exposure to a contagious disease, especially chicken pox or mumps
- fever or any sign of infection that persists or worsens
- persistent headaches
- redness or inflammation in certain areas of the body
- eyesight problems (blurred or double vision)
- unexpected vomiting, especially if not linked to irradiation or chemotherapy

This list is limited to major problems. Your doctor will discuss other potential problems with you. If in doubt, always ask for advice.

Conclusion

Recovering from an illness is never easy; it takes patience, determination, and a great deal of courage.

Understanding your body, its defense mechanisms, and the diseases that affect it is a crucial step in any course of treatment. The time when patients waited passively to be cured, stretched out on hospital beds like puppets at the end of solute lines, is long past in my view. We are living in an era of communications, an era when people hunger for knowledge. If patients are not given adequate information, inevitably they will look elsewhere for answers and, unfortunately, what they are told is often biased. Patients may even lose confidence and delay a treatment. Taking an active part in treatment and understanding the illness can help patients to achieve recovery and can make them aware of habits and lifestyles that may be harmful.

Recently, a forty-four-year-old man—father to a young family, a businessman who loved to eat and smoked heavily, a patient who was diagnosed with coronary disease and needed a triple bypass—told me: "Doctor, I can't wait for my operation to be over and done with—I'll be cured at last."

But surgery is only one step in recovery; much more subtle, and requiring just as much courage on the part of the patient, is a second type of intervention, and it is vital. If the patient does not eliminate certain specific habits, the heart bypass will be purely palliative.

The factors underlying malignant blood diseases and cancers are certainly not as well known as those that lead to coronary disease, but awareness of one's body and one's habits and lifestyle are every bit as important in both instances.

This second type of intervention can extend beyond our individual lifestyles. As we have seen, several environmental factors can affect our health. Some people claim that being aware of these problems is a source of stress in itself, but the contrary can be true as well. All agree, however, that access to accurate information can only be in everyone's best interests.

I hope that those who have a malignant disease and who have read this book have found the answers to some of their questions; I hope this book has sparked their curiosity. To each of you, I say: Never be reluctant to ask your doctor for details on your illness. Now that you know more about it, move on with your life and, above all else, never lose hope.

Since I had my bone marrow transplant; I have

- finished my medical studies;
- worked as an ER doctor for the last 10 years;
- run two marathons;
- climbed Mount Blanc (France), Mount Kilimanjaro (Kenya), and Mount Aconcagua (Argentina);
- finished two ocean sailboating races, one across the Atlantic and two in Newport, Bermuda, in 1998 and 1999.

And I still have a lot more to do.

Dr. Robert Patenaude

Glossary of Medical Terms Used in Oncology

Adenocarcinoma: type of cancer beginning in glandular tissues (microscopic glands); it is found mainly in the lungs, the digestive tract and the pancreas.

AIDS (acquired immunodeficiency syndrome): a serious infectious disease that can be transmitted sexually or through the blood (blood transfusion, needles, etc.). AIDS is caused by a virus that penetrates the lymphocytes and prevents them from fighting diseases. AIDS patients are sensitive to several germs, described as opportunistic, which do not affect healthy individuals.

New drugs and vaccines are currently under study and by all indications, in a few years it will be possible to control this disease.

Allogenic bone marrow transplant: a bone marrow transplant where the patient receives bone marrow from another individual. We designate the donor by the term "related" if she or he is a sister or brother of the patent; the term "unrelated" designates a donor who comes from an international bone marrow registry.

Alopecia: loss of hair, often associated with anticancer treatments (*see also* Baldness).

Anatomy: representation of the human body and its main organs.

Androgens: hormones responsible for male characteristics (a deep voice, beard, sexual characteristics).

Anemia: blood disease characterized by a decrease in the number of red blood cells or the hemoglobin level and leading to a state of weakness and exhaustion.

Antibiotic: a drug used to fight infections; it can be administered orally, intravenously, by local application, in the form of drops or salves for the eyes, ears, and skin.

Antibody: small particles that have the property of sticking in a particular way to a given antigen. Antibodies are part of the human immune system; they fight infections and play a major role in rejection reactions.

Anticancer or antineoplastic: refers to chemical or biological substances used in the treatment of cancer. Anticancer or cytotoxic substances prevent cells from dividing and thus, prevent tumors from growing. However, they never destroy a tumor completely, which results in the need to use several anticancer drugs at once, over prolonged periods of time; this is known as a treatment program (*see also* Chemotherapy and Chapter 5).

Antigens: small structures found on the surface of cells and foreign bodies such as viruses and bacteria. These structures have the property of stimulating the formation of antibodies.

Anti-lymphocytic globulins (ATGs): antibodies directed against lymphocytic type white cells. These globulins are particularly effective in the treatment of aplastic anemia.

Apheresis: a techniques used to withdraw certain blood cells or blood constituents. Apheresis is used to collect blood cells and stem cells (cytopheresis) and plasma (plasmapheresis).

Aplastic anemia: a serious disease characterized by a disappearance of stem cells in the bone marrow. The blood becomes poor in red and white blood cells and platelets (*see* Chapter 4).

Artifact: disturbance in the result of a biological or radiological examination caused by an error in the use of a technique. For example, the reading of a bone marrow sample can by falsified because a specimen has not been spread properly on the slide or because the sample has coagulated before being spread on the slide. As the result of an artifact, the doctor must take a new sample.

Arteries: vessels bringing blood pumped by the heart to all parts of the body (*see* "The Cardiorespiratory System," pages 68–69).

Ascites: an accumulation of liquid in the stomach. The causes of ascites are improper functioning of the liver, the heart, and the kidneys, and the presence of certain types of cancer.

Asepsis: a method of grouping together several techniques designed to prevent the introduction of germs that could infect the immunosuppressed patient. During a bone marrow transplant, the air in the patient's room is filtered and floors and walls are disinfected daily. Visitors are asked to wash their hands and to wear a lab coat and a surgical mask. Food is even cooked at high temperatures. These precautions are used to decrease the risk of infection.

Aspergillosis: an infection of the bronchi and the lungs by aspergillus. The microscopic fungi affect mainly immunosuppressed patients. The infection can become very severe and, therefore, must be treated quickly using antibiotics that are administered intravenously.

Aspergillus: a microscopic fungi.

Autograft: the autograft or autologous graft is a graft in which the patient acts as his or her own donor.

Autologous bone marrow transplant: a bone marrow transplant where the patient is his or her own donor.

Bacteria: very small organisms that are visible only through a microscope. Bacteria can be rounded in shape, in which case they are known as "cocci," or they can look like elongated sticks, in which case they are known as "bacillae." Bacteria can cause several types of infections, the most common of which are pneumonia, bronchitis, urinary infections, gastroenteritis, meningitis, catheter infections, and bed sores.

To identify bacteria accurately, samples must be taken directly from the site of the infection.

If the site of the infection is unknown and if the patient suffers from a high fever, bacteriemia (the presence of bacteria in the blood) is a likely diagnosis; blood samples are taken through repeated venous punctures (hemocultures).

Identifying bacteria in a laboratory can take several days.

The doctor will prescribe antibiotics immediately, and when the bacteria have been identified, will readjust the treatment to destroy them as effectively as possible.

Glossary

Baldness: an absence of hair on the skull. During chemotherapy treatments, patients may suffer from temporary hair loss, since hair growth is linked to a rapid multiplication of the dermis's cells, which are very sensitive to anticancer treatments.

Basophiles: white cells belonging to the polynuclear family, capable of absorbing blue dyes.

Benign cells: cells that can form a small tumor, but that do not have the invasive nature of malignant cells. Such tumors are benign and, therefore, pose no immediate threat to a patient's health.

Biochemistry: the science that studies the natural chemical reactions, basic in all human beings.

Biology: the science that studies living things (vegetable, animal, and human) at all stages of their development.

Biopsy: a sampling of fragments of certain organs, taken for microscopic examination. The most common biopsies are biopsies of the skin, the bones, the liver, and the lungs. The biopsy makes it possible to arrive at an accurate diagnosis of a disease.

Blasts: young cells, the precursors of white cells, red cells, and platelets. These "baby" cells mature in the bone marrow and they are full grown, the leave the marrow, entering the blood in the form of mature cells. Blasts are found solely in the bone marrow. Their presence in the blood is unusual; when they are detected in the blood, doctors look for serious infections, an inflammatory disease, a hemorrhage and, at times, leukemia or another form of cancer affecting the bone marrow.

Blood coagulation: a reaction in which the blood forms a clot to stop a hemorrhage (*see* "Blood Clot Formation," page 63).

Blood culture: a bacteria culture that consists of a blood sample taken by venous culture. The blood culture makes it possible to identify the type of bacteria that has infiltrated the blood, causing septicemia. Usually, to increase the chances of isolating the germs, three blood samples are taken through punctures made at two or three different sites.

Blood group: there are several blood group systems, the best-known being the ABO system.

On their surface, an individual's red cells carry small particles (antigens) that belong to Group A or Group B or, if they belong to both groups, the AB group.

If they have no type, they are referred to as Group O.

If the individual belongs to Group A, his or her serum contains antibodies against Group B, called the anti-B antibody; this is why he or she must receive transfusions of blood that belongs to Group B or Group AB.

Table Representing the ABO Blood Group System

Subject's blood group	Antibodies present	Blood group used should the subject require a transfusion
Group A	Anti-B	Group A Group O
Group B	Anti-A	Group B Group O
Group AB	None	Group A Group B Group O
Group O	Anti-A Anti-B	Group O

Similarly, a subject from Group B cannot receive a blood transfusion from Group A or AB, since it contains anti-A antibodies.

Subjects in Group AB have no anti-A or anti-B antibodies, so they are universal recipients.

Subjects from Group O have both types of antibodies in their serum; they can receive blood solely from Group O. However, since their red cells have no A and B antigens, these subjects can give their blood to anyone, regardless of whether they belong to Group A, B, or AB; they are universal donors.

During a bone marrow transplant, the blood groups of the donor and the recipient are a major concern.

Bronchi: semi-rigid conduits designed to transport air between the trachea and pulmonary alveoli.

Bronchitis: an infection of the bronchi. Its symptoms are coughing, spitting and, at times, fever.

Bronchoscopy: an examination making it possible to observe the lower part of the trachea and the bronchi. Bronchoscopy is a short examination and it requires only a local anesthetic to desensitize the throat; the examination is done through a flexible tube of small diameter.

Bruising: the accumulation of blood under the skin, usually caused by a traumatism. A spontaneous bruise is red in color, then successively becoming blue, greenish, and pale yellow; it disappears within three weeks.

Bulsufan: a drug used in chemotherapy, in tablet form, particularly effective against chronic leukemias. Its side effects are sterility, an increase in skin pigmentation, a drying of mucous membranes, and pulmonary fibrosis.

Cachexia: a state of extreme emaciation observed in the terminal phase of some cancers, or starvation.

Caloric needs: the calories needed for the proper functioning of all of the body's organs. Caloric needs are based on the individual's weight and size. The need increases during physical activity, in the post-treatment phase, in the post-operative phase, and when the patient presents a graft versus host (GVH) reaction of an infection.

Cancer: the anarchic proliferation of cells described as malignant, which at their original site form a malignant lump or tumor. The malignant cells can spread and can lead to the formation of metastases.

Cancerous resistance: a phenomenon according to which cancerous cells become resistant to a given form of chemotherapy.

Candida albicans: micro-organisms that are part of microscopic fungi that in their natural state, live in the mucous membranes, principally the vagina, the nose, and the mouth.

Candidiasis, also named moniliasis, is a candida infection that can result from the ingestion of antibiotics or a weakening of the immune system. In most cases, candidiasis is a harmless infection (for example, candidiasis in the mouth of a child who is taking antibiotics). However, in patients who have undergone immunosuppression, it can lead to pneumonia or septicemia, both of which may be severe.

Carcinogenic: a factor that causes cancer. For example, smoking causes cancer of the larynx, the lungs, and the esophagus.

Carcinoma: a cancer which begins on the surface of certain organs. Carcinoma of the skin, or skin cancer, is among the most common forms.

Carbon dioxide: a gas produced by the work of cells in all human organs. Carbon dioxide is absorbed by red cells, which transport it to the lungs, which release it into the air.

Catheter: a small, thin plastic tube that can be introduced into a vein, an artery, or any cavity from which liquid must be removed; it is also used to administer drugs.

Cell: the smallest living structure in our organism. Several cells grouped together and fulfilling a very specific function form an organ. Thus, the liver, the lungs, the brain, the heart, the muscles, the bone marrow, and all other organs in our body, without exception, are composed of cells. In the case of the blood, we sometimes use the term corpuscle, a synonym for cell (*see* "The Cell," Chapter 2).

Central nervous system: an expression used to describe the brain and cerebrospinal fluid.

Centrifugation: the action of using very rapid movement to separate elements of different density from one another; for example, the various types of blood cells.

Cerebrospinal fluid: the clear liquid that circulates in the spinal column (*see* Lumbar Puncture), surrounding the spinal cord and the brain.

Chemotherapy: the treatment of cancer through chemical or biological agents that act on the cells to prevent them from multiplying. Some drugs enter the nucleus, others enter the cytoplasm; they are designed to block the cell's functions. The combination of several drugs acting on different sites leads to a more extensive destruction of cancerous cells. This method of treatment is known as polychemotherapy. These drugs are not specific to cancerous cells; they also inhibit the multiplication of any cell that divides rapidly. The capillary cells of hair and the intestine's cells are particularly sensitive because they divide rapidly, which explains the hair loss and decrease in intestinal absorption observed during treatments.

Glossary

Chloroma: a very rare form of leukemia found in children, characterized by greenish tumors on the skin.

Chromosomes: small stick-like bodies located in the nuclei of cells. Chromosomes are visible under a microscope during cell division.They contain all of the cell's genes; by dividing in pairs, chromosomes transmit genes from one cell to another. Humans have twenty-three pairs of chromosomes.

Clinical stage: an expression that designates by letters or numbers the degree to which a disease has progressed. For some diseases, such as Hodgkin's disease, the clinical stage determines the type of treatment program that will be used.

Clot: a gelatinous mass resulting from the blood's coagulation. The clot is formed of platelets, red cells, and proteins and its main function is to stop hemorrhaging.

Contraindication: a circumstance or a period of time in which the patient's condition makes it dangerous or even impossible to begin a treatment program or to administer a drug.

Corpuscle: a blood cell. There are red corpuscles and white corpuscles (*see* Cell).

Corticotherapy: a treatment based on synthetic or natural hormones, the most common of which is cortisone.

Its biological actions are multiple; it is used as an antirejection agent because it is very effective in diminishing the immune system's action (*see* Immunosuppression). It also has an anticancer effect and therefore is used in several polychemotherapy treatment programs. It also has an anti-inflammatory effect, which makes it useful in the treatment of diseases such as rheumatoid arthritis, inflammatory diseases of the intestines, and collagen-related diseases. Corticotherapy has certain side effects: it increases fatty tissues, which causes weight gain and causes the face to appear swollen. Over the long term, it can lead to diabetes, high blood pressure, and osteoporosis. In some instances, other drugs are used to counter these side effects. When corticotherapy is stopped, all side effects disappear rapidly.

Cortisone: *see* Corticotherapy.

Curative treatment: a form of treatment whose objective is to cure the patient.

Cyclosporin: a mushroom extract, this drug is one of the most commonly used in various organ transplants and in bone marrow transplants involving a donor. It is very effective in stopping rejection reactions and the graft versus host reaction. The drug's principle side effects are high blood pressure and an increase in hair growth. These effects disappear when the patient stops taking cyclosporin.

Cyst: a cavity surrounded by a liquid-containing wall. Generally, cysts are benign and can be removed surgically.

Cystitis: an inflammation of the bladder, usually caused by an infection or an anticancer drug. The patient complains of pain when urinating and in some instances the urine takes on a pinkish color. Although unpleasant, cystitis is a temporary condition and is easy to treat. If it is associated with fever, we have to suspect kidney infection (pyelonephritis).

Cytogenetics: the study of genetics on the cellular level.

Cytomegalovirus: a virus often designated by the abbreviation CMV. This virus is common in the general population. In a healthy individual, the infection takes the form of a common cold. Subsequently, the virus remains in the blood in a latent form, for the rest of the individual's life. In contrast, patients suffering from immunosuppression experience high fevers and, at times, pneumonia and hepatitis, both of which can be very severe. Cytomegalovirus infections are treated with antibiotics.

Cytopheresis: a process which consists of separating the various types of cells (red and white cells, platelets) from other blood components (plasma) by centrifugation (*see* Apheresis) and collecting them.

Cytotoxic: a term used to describe a drug that is toxic for the cells.

Diagnosis: the determination of the exact nature of a disease.

Differential diagnosis: a comparison between the diagnosis made by the doctor and the diseases that involve similar symptoms.

Dietician: an individual specialized in the development of nutritional programs that meet the patient's caloric needs.

Diuretic: a drug that causes an increase in the quantity of urine excreted by the patient. For example, furosemide is a powerful diuretic.

DNA: a complex substance that at the molecular level resembles a long helix. DNA is found in chromosomes and is responsible for inherited traits (*see* "The Cell").

Glossary

Dry bone marrow puncture: a puncture that fails to collect liquid. A dry bone marrow puncture is linked to certain diseases such as aplasia, myelofibrosis, and some leukemias.

Early menopause: menopause that occurs before the usual age; it may result from a gynecological problem. During anticancer treatments, it is often caused by chemotherapy or radiotherapy, which produce ovarian failure. In such instances, a hormone-based treatment is administered and continues until young patients have reached the age of fifty-five to sixty.

Edema: the swelling of an organ caused by an accumulation of liquid; for example, patients suffering from renal or heart failure often experience a swelling of the legs.

Embolism: an obliteration of a blood vessel, either arterial or venous, by a foreign body or substance (a blood clot, a fatty body, air, bacteria). The sites most commonly affected are the lungs, the brain, or the arteries in lower limbs.

Endocarditis: a serious infection affecting the inner heart, where heart valves are found.

Endocrinology: a science focussing on the study of the glands and the hormones they secrete. Diabetes militus is a well-known disease that is studied and treated by endocrinologists.

Endometrium: the inner portion of the cavity of the uterus.

Enteritis: an inflammation of the small intestine, often associated with a stomach infection (gastroenteritis). Its symptoms are diarrhea, nausea, and vomiting.

Enzymes: proteins used in the chemical reaction of cells. Some enzymes are secreted outside the cell; for example, digestion is a complex process requiring several enzymes secreted by the pancreas.

Erythropoietin: This is a natural substance used to increase the bone marrow's production of red cells.

This messenger is manufactured in large quantity by the kidneys. Since the kidneys are very sensitive to drops in oxygen levels and to anemia, they react to the slightest decrease in the number of red cells by manufacturing erythropoietin. The secretion of erythropoietin incites the bone marrow to manufacture red cells in large numbers.

The use of synthetic erythropoietin (eprex) makes it possible to correct anemia while decreasing the number of blood transfusions; this drug is particularly useful for patients suffering from several renal insufficiencies.

Esophagus: the first part of the digestive tract linking the mouth to the stomach.

Esophagitis: an inflammation of the esophagus that may result from anticancer treatments, an infection (for example, a candidiasis) or a GVH reaction.

Ewing's sarcoma: a cancer found mainly in adolescents. It usually begins in long bones, especially the tibia and the femur. Young patients complain of bone pain, excessive fatigue caused by anemia, and excessive sweating.

Until recently, Ewing's sarcoma was an incurable cancer; new treatment programs now result in a recovery rate of 75 percent among patients who present no metastases.

Failure: the impossibility for an organ or a gland to fulfill its normal functions.

Fanconi's anemia: serious congenital disease which, in addition to anemia, involves a decrease in white cells and platelets. The disease may also involve malformations of the bones and kidneys and at times, dark spots on the skin (see "Congenital Diseases of the Blood System," page 149).

Fever (hyperthermia): an abnormal rise in body temperature, accompanied by general discomfort. At rest, the body's normal temperature is approximately 98.6°F (37.5°C).

Some factors such as physical exercise, pregnancy, or ovulation can raise the body's temperature, but this phenomenon is not described as a fever.

Apart from the above-mentioned examples, an increase in temperature is the body's reaction to an aggression, most often infectious in nature.

Fibrosis: a thickening of a tissue or an organ as a reaction against an aggressive factor; an organ affected by fibrosis is gradually replaced by hard tissue and its functioning is diminished.

Foreign body: a substance that is foreign to the organism and that comes from outside the organism, such as a projectile or an object, a virus, a bacterium, or an insertion in part of an organ (artificial heart valve) or a whole organ (kidney, heart, lung, liver, or pancreas transplant). In instances involving the transplanting of whole organs, if the immune system recognizes the organ as foreign, a rejection reaction ensues.

Full-body irradiation: exposure of all parts of the body to rays. Full-body irradiation is sometimes used in radiotherapy before a bone marrow transplant.

Furosemide (Lasix): a drug used to increase the formation of urine in the kidneys.

Gammaglobulin: a term describing all antibodies contained in the blood. Globulins can be extracted from a normal person's blood serum by plasmapheresis and can be transfused into a patient suffering from an antibody deficiency.

Ganglion or lymph node: located along vessels known as lymphatic caniculi, founding throughout the human body. Ganglions can easily be felt in the neck, armpits and groin. Ganglions contain white cells known as lymphocytes.

When an infection is present, these cells multiply in the ganglions located near the site of the infection; in turn, this causes a swelling of the ganglions, a condition that last for a few weeks. Ganglions can also increase in size if they are affected by cancer, in which case they are known as lymphomas. At times, they can be the site of metastases caused by a cancer affecting an adjacent organ.

Gastritis: an inflammation of the wall of the stomach, caused by excessive acidity.

Gastroenteritis: *see* Enteritis.

Gastroenterology: the science that studies the intestine and other organs involved in digestive mechanisms.

General anesthetic: a technique used to sedate patients who must undergo surgery.

Genetics: the science that studies heredity.

Germs: a general term used to describe all viruses, bacteria, and microscopic fungi.

Glioblastoma: cancer of the nervous system.

Glucose: a sugar that is one of the body's main sources of energy.

Glycoproteins: molecules grouping together a glucide (sugar) and a protide (protein). Glycoproteins are found on the surface of red blood cells and form the antigens that correspond to certain blood groups.

Graft: bone marrow taken from an individual for transplant purposes; the usual quantity is between 500 and 1,000 cubic centimeters. The term graft can also designate other types of organs (for example, in the case of a heart transplant, the heart is referred to as a graft).

Graft versus Host (GVH): a rejection reaction specific to a bone marrow transplant, in which grafted cells (grafts) attack the recipient (host or patient).

Unlike the usual rejection phenomenon in which the recipient's immune system rejects the transplanted organ (for example, rejection of a kidney or heart transplant), if a GVH reaction occurs following a bone marrow transplant, the donor's immune system attacks the recipient of the graft.

Graft versus Leukemia (GVL): a phenomenon under which grafted cells (grafts) attack leukemic cells that may survive even after a transplant. This reaction is linked to the graft versus host reaction.

Granulocyte: the name given to certain white cells whose nuclei contain several lobes. The word granulocyte is a synonym of polynuclear (*see* Chapter 2).

GVH: *see* Graft versus Host.

Hematopoiesis: the formation of blood cells (white and red cells and platelets); in humans, hematopoiesis takes place mainly in the bone marrow, but also in the liver and spleen.

Hematopoietic growth factors or cell colony stimulation factors: natural substances manufactured by the organism, causing the stem cells in bone marrow to multiply. Growth factors are now available in drug form. GM-CSF (granulocyte megacaryocyte colony stimulating factor) causes stem cells to produce white cells of the granulocytic type; it is used after chemotherapy to make white cells reappear more quickly, thus reducing the risk of opportunistic infections.

Erythropoietin is also a growth factor, stimulating the manufacture of red cells; it is administered to patients suffering from renal failure, to reduce anemia.

Glossary

Hematology: the science that studies the blood and blood diseases.

Hemodialysis: a technique using a sophisticated piece of equipment known as a dialyzer, used to cleanse blood of certain accumulated impurities, usually excreted by the kidneys. Hemodialysis is very useful for patients suffering from severe kidney disease.

Hemoglobin: a bright red substance that gives red cells their characteristic color. Hemoglobin transports oxygen and carbon dioxide between the lungs and all of the body's other organs. Among women, the normal hemoglobin level is approximately 130 grams per liter; among men, it is approximately 140 grams per liter. When the hemoglobin level drops, the condition is known as anemia.

Hemolysis: the destruction of red cells. There is a natural hemolysis of red cells when they reach the end of their life cycle (120 days).

In certain instances (serious infections, intoxication with lead or arsenic, the ingestion of certain drugs, the presence of a mechanical heart valve, the consequences of a blood transfusion, the presence of other diseases such as leukemias, lymphomas and inflammatory diseases), hemolysis can be major and can cause jaundice and anemia (hemolytic anemia). Therefore, it is always important to find the cause of hemolysis and to treat it quickly.

Hemorrhage: loss of blood from a blood-containing vessel.

Heparin: a substance that prevents blood coagulation.

Hepatic: a term used to describe any phenomenon related to the liver. For example, a hepatic biopsy s a liver biopsy.

Hepatitis: a liver disease caused by toxic substances (toxic hepatitis) or a virus (viral hepatitis).

Heredity: a term describing the method of transmission to descendants of certain physical characteristics and diseases.

HIV (Human Immunodeficiency Virus): a term used to describe the AIDS virus.

HLA (Human Leucocytic Antigen): a term designating the antigens located on the white cells that are responsible for compatibility in cases involving transplants.

Hodgkin's disease or Hodgkin's lymphoma: a cancerous disease located in the ganglions (lymph nodes) but also found in other organs such as the liver, the spleen, the lungs, and the nervous system.

General symptoms include fever, weight loss, and a swelling of the nodes. Always fatal in the past, the prognosis for this disease has improved considerably thanks to chemotherapy and radiotherapy treatments and bone marrow transplants. Currently, the recovery rate is higher than 90 percent (*see* "Lymphomas," page 137).

Hormones: substances manufactured by certain glands and travelling in the blood toward other organs and tissues, where they fulfill their functions. There are hundreds of hormones, divided into three main categories, as shown in the following table:

Main Hormones and Their Functions

Hormones	Functions
1. Steroid hormones (Cortisone)	• Plays a role in reactions to physical stress (hemorrhaging, burns, surgical procedures, etc.).
(Testosterone)	• Is responsible for male characteristics in humans, such as pilosity (beard, chest hair) and the breaking of the voice, and female characteristics (breast development, the menstrual cycle, and pregnancy).
2. Hormones manufactured by the pancreas (Insulin)	• Decreases the sugar concentration found in the blood.
3. Hormones that act on the cardiovascular system (Adrenaline)	• Increases the heart beat rate and blood pressure, dilates the bronchi, and increases the concentration of sugars in the blood.
Thyroid hormone	• Stabilizes weight, the heart beat rate, intestinal functions, and the individual's energy level.

Glossary

Hormonotherapy: a hormone-based treatment designed to counter a lack. For example, in the case of menopause, patients are given replacement hormones.

HVG (Host versus Graft): a term used to describe the reaction in which a recipient rejects a transplanted organ; for example, the rejection of a kidney subsequent to a kidney transplant, or rejection of a bone marrow transplant.

Hydrocephalus: an increase in the perimeter of the skull in children. Caused by an obstruction in the flow of cerebrospinal fluid, the problem results from several diseases, including osteopetrosis, spina bifida, and some infections and tumors. To prevent neurological complications, hydrocephalus must be treated quickly.

Hydroxyurea: a drug used in chemotherapy treatment programs, mainly to fight chronic leukemias. The drug is administered in tablet form and has few side effects.

Hyperthermia: *see* Fever. It occurs when the temperature of the body exceeds 98.6°F or 37.5°C.

Idiosyncratic effect: a expression used to describe a hypersensitivity to a given drug, regardless of the dose administered.

Iliac: upper part of the pelvis, where bone marrow is particularly rich in stem cells. The iliac is readily accessible and therefore is a prime site for bone marrow punctures.

Immunity: the phenomenon of the body's resistance to an infectious disease.

Immunodeficiency or immunosuppression: the immune system's inability to fight infections. The immune system is composed of several types of white cells whose function is to destroy the infectious agents that enter our bodies. A person can become immunosuppressed temporarily during anticancer treatments such as high-dose chemotherapies and radiotherapy. For example, in the case of a bone marrow transplant, approximately three to six weeks are required before the transplant recipient has a sufficient number of white cells to function in a normal environment. To avoid the risk of infection, he or she must wear a surgical mask for 120 days. If a GVH occurs, the patient must take certain anti-rejection drugs that may also decrease the immune system's effectiveness.

Immunodeficiencies are also found in newborns, in the form of congenital diseases (agammaglobulinemia). These diseases are sometimes linked to hematological diseases such as leukemias, lymphomas, myelomas, and aplastic anemias.

Some severe infections can decrease our resistance; AIDS is a well-known example.

Patients suffering from immunodeficiency are more susceptible to infections, the most common of which are gastroenteritis, sinusitis, and pneumonia.

Infectious agents which thrive on the weakness in an individual's defence mechanisms are known as opportunistic germs. The most common are candida albicans, aspergillus, cytomegalovirus, pneumocystosis and tuberculosis.

Fortunately, new antibiotics are effective in treating most of these infections.

Immunology: the study of immunity and resulting reactions. Immunology studies the mechanisms that enable the body to fight infections, allergies, rejection reactions, and the development of certain cancers.

Immunosuppression: a synonym for immunodeficiency.

Immunosuppressive: a term used to describe a treatment or a disease that decreases an individual's immunity.

Immunotherapy: a treatment designed to increase immunity to fight a disease; for example, a new drug called interferon increases the body's immunity and prevents the further development of certain cancers.

Incidence: the number of new cases of a given disease, in a given population group, over a fixes period of time.

Incompatibility: the impossibility for certain elements to coexist.

Induction: the initial phase of a treatment program, designed to achieve a remission of the disease.

Infection: the overall modifications in the organism (fever, sweating, coughing, fatigue, etc.) resulting from a bacterium that has penetrated our body. If the infection is local, the bacterium is confined to the tissue it penetrates, as is the case with a skin infection resulting from a dirty wound.

But the infection can go beyond the first defense mechanisms (the skin, the lymph nodes, the mouth, the throat, and the tonsils) and can

spread to adjacent organs; for example, a bacterium responsible for ton-
sillitis can spread to the lungs, can cause bronchitis and even pneumonia.
It can sometimes spread to the blood (septicemia) and several other
organs (liver, kidneys, the nervous system, joints, etc.).

Inflammation: the reactions caused by an aggression, which define its nature
(burns, contusions, insect bites, infections, etc.). The inflammatory reaction is characterized by pain, redness, and warmth near the site of the
aggression.

Inflammatory diseases: diseases whose main characteristic is to produce
inflammation in certain parts of the body. Arthritis is an inflammatory
disease affecting the joints.

Interferon: a substance produced by certain cells in our bodies. Interferon
is a natural way of increasing our immunity and it helps fight infections.
For the past several years, interferon has been manufactured in laboratories and it is used to control the development of certain leukemias
(hairy cell leukemia, chronic myelogenous leukemia, and myeloma)
and other cancers.

Interleukin: a substance produced by the macrophages and other white corpuscles.

There are numerous subcategories of interleukin (Interleukins I to …).
In the course of immune system reactions, these substances play a
major role as messengers. They increase the multiplication of lymphocytes that stimulate the bone marrow and result in fevers when infections are present.

On the therapeutic level, they are the focus of intense research.
Recently, scientists discovered that they allow the multiplication of lymphocytes specialized in the recognition and destruction of certain types
of cancer.

Tests conducted by Dr. Rosenberg in skin cancer (melanoma) cases
are very promising and pave the way to a new form of treatment.

Intolerance: the body's intense and abnormal reaction to a drug. For example,
a person who cannot tolerate penicillin can experience severe nausea and,
at times, vomiting; on the other hand, most individuals have no reaction to this particular antibiotic.

Irradiation: exposure to ultraviolet or radioactive rays (*see* Radiotherapy).

Ischemia: a decrease in the blood flow to a given part of the body; if the decrease persists, it will involve lesions in certain organs in the "ischemic" region. For example, when there is an obstruction in one of the coronary arteries bringing blood to the heart, there is "cardiac ischemia"; if the obstruction persists, there is a lesion of the cardiac muscle or an "infarction."

Isogenic donor: a term used to describe a donor who is the identical twin of a patient.

Jaundice: a yellow coloring of the skin. Generally, jaundice is caused by liver disease; more rarely, it is the result of hemolysis of red cells.

Kaposi's sarcoma: a cancer of the skin characterized by a violet-tinged red coloring. Kaposi's sarcoma is often linked with AIDS.

Keratitis: a painful inflammation of the cornea; often caused by the herpes virus.

Laparoscopy: an examination practiced in an operating room, with the patient under general anesthetic. A rigid tube (laparoscope) is introduced into the abdomen, making it possible for the doctor to observe various organs in the abdominal cavity, such as the liver, the ovaries, the appendix, and the kidneys. The laparoscopy is very useful in confirming the diagnosis of certain diseases of the abdomen, such as appendicitis, ectopic pregnancies, and ovarian cysts.

Laparotomy: abdominal surgery carried under general anesthetic, in an operating room. The doctor makes a small incision in the abdomen to evaluate the condition of internal organs (the ovaries, the appendix, lymph nodes, the liver, the spleen, the pancreas, and the intestines), to verify the extent of a disease or to proceed with biopsies required to arrive at a diagnosis.

Lasix (furosemide): a drug used to increase the formation of urine in the kidneys.

Lesion: an alteration of a tissue or an organ, caused by a disease or a traumatism.

Lethal: a term used to describe something fatal.

Leukemia: cancer of the white cells. For more details on various types of leukemia, *see* Chapter 4.

Leucocytes: a synonym for white cells.

Glossary

Leucocyte concentration: an increase in the number of white cells. Leucocyte concentration can result from an infection, an inflammation, or leukemia.

Leukopenia: a decrease in the number of white cells. Leukopenia can result from the early stages of an infection, from aplasia, or from leukemia.

Lipids: a term used to describe the fats contained in our blood, the most well-known of which are cholesterol and triglycerides.

Local: limited to a small part of an organ or a tissue.

Local anesthetic: a technique involving a subcutaneous injection, used to make a particular area of the body insensitive to pain.

Lumbar puncture: a technique used to collect cerebrospinal fluid to analyze its contents and arrive at a diagnosis.

After local anesthetic, the doctor introduces a fine needle between two lumbar vertebrae, reaching the cerebrospinal fluid and collecting a few cubic centimeters.

In the case of a cancer investigation, the presence of cancerous cells in the fluid indicates that the disease has spread to the nervous system. In the case of an investigation related to an infection, the presence of a high number of white cells and bacteria indicates a infection of the cerebrospinal fluid (meningitis).

A lumbar puncture can be used to introduce certain drugs (chemotherapy drugs, antibiotics) into the patient's system, to fight the disease.

Lymph: a whitish liquid composed of white cells (lymphocytes) and nutritional substances, circulating in the lymphatic vessels.

Lymphadenopathy: a term used to describe lymph nodes that have increased in size. The increase in size can be caused by infections, some diseases, and some forms of cancer.

Lymphatic: the small vessels contained in the lymph that runs through the body and connects nodes to one another.

Lymphatic vessels play a major role in the body's immune system since the white cells (lymphocytes) use them to travel to the nodes, where they multiple if an infection is present.

At times, malignant cells leave a primary cancer site and spread to lymphatic vessels, infiltrating surrounding nodes. For example, breast cancer often leads to metastases in the nodes found in the armpit.

236

Lymphocytes: a type of white cells with a large, circular nucleus. When an infection occurs, lymphocytes multiply in the lymph nodes and attack the germs. There are many types of lymphocytes, each of which has a specific job to do. For example, Type B lymphocytes manufacture antibodies. The AIDS virus attacks lymphocytes and prevents them from fighting bacteria, which explains why AIDS patients are vulnerable to infectious agents.

Lymphoma: cancer of the lymph nodes. See Chapter 4.

Lysosomes: small microscopic spheres consisting of a lipid (oily) matter and capable of containing drugs. Lysosomes are used experimentally in certain chemotherapy treatment programs; they have the advantage of penetrating cancerous cells more easily.

Macrophages: white cells whose main role is to digest certain particles (cellular wastes, foreign bodies, etc.).

Malignancy: the tendency for a disease to progress toward a form of cancer.

Malignant cells: cells that have become cancerous; they multiply nonstop and eventually invade adjacent organs. These cells can also form tumors, which are described as malignant.

Melanoma: a very serious cancer of the skin, often originating in a nevus (type of freckle) that increases in size and takes on a black- or blue-tinged color. A freckle that changes in size and color should be examined immediately by a doctor. Early diagnosis is very important since melanomas are aggressive and quickly lead to metastases.

The treatment of choice is surgery. If metastases are present at diagnosis or if they appear a few months subsequent to the disease's onset, radiotherapy, chemotherapy, or both forms of treatment will be required.

Unfortunately, melanoma can sometimes be very resistant to conventional treatments. New treatments such as immunotherapy and autologous bone marrow transplants are the focus of experiments, and preliminary results are promising.

Molecular biology: the science that studies the internal mechanism that are responsible for the proper functioning and the multiplication of cells. Molecular biology focuses more particularly on the reactions that occur in the nucleus of the cell.

Meningitis: an infection of the cerebrospinal fluid surrounding the brain and the spinal cord. The patient suffers from intense headaches, a high fever, and pain in the spinal column when bending. Meningitis cases must be diagnosed quickly using lumbar puncture; the disease can be fatal if not treated immediately.

Menopause: a definite stoppage in menstruation; menopause occurs between the ages of forty-five and fifty-five. Symptoms include irregular menstrual cycles, fatigue, and hot flashes.

Metabolism: the biological changes that occur within our body's cells.

Metastasis (See Color Plate No. 15): a cancerous site that has developed outside the original site of the primary cancer. For example, cancer cells originating in the intestines are often found in the liver. In such instances, doctors refer to liver metastases originating from an intestinal cancer. Often, metastases cause more problems than a primary cancer; for example, a melanoma or skin cancer becomes very serious if it leads to metastases of the brain. We often use the term "generalized cancer" to describe the situation where several organs are affected by metastases.

Microbiology: the science that studies various infectious agents, their means of spreading, and their treatment.

Mononucleosis: a benign infectious disease caused by a virus. This disease occurs mainly among adolescents, who suffer from sore throats, fatigue and fever. Upon examination, the doctor discovers that the lymph nodes in the neck have increased in size. This disease is often referred to as the "kissing disease" of teenagers. The only risk linked with mononucleosis is an increase in the size of the spleen, which can persist for up to two months; a swollen spleen is fragile since it may rupture and lead to an abdominal hemorrhage. Consequently, patients suffering from mononucleosis must avoid all forms of violent sports.

Morphine: a drug used to decrease pain levels (analgesic). Its repeated use leads to habituation, in which case doses must be increased regularly to obtain effective pain relief.

Mucositis: an inflammation of the mouth causing a burning sensation.

Mutation: the transformation of a cell's gene, possibly making it cancerous. The causes underlying mutation are radiation, viruses and come chemical substances (*see* Cancer).

Mutism: a refusal to speak.

Mycosis: an infection of the skin by certain microscopic fungi. In severe cases of immunodeficiency, other organs can also be affected (lungs, intestines, liver).

Nausea: a discomfort often associated with chemotherapy treatment programs; fortunately, several medications (Gravol, Stemetil, Maxeran) are effective in countering nausea.

Nephroblastoma (Wilms tumor): a cancer most frequently found in children aged young than five years. Generally, parents consult their doctors because they have noticed that their child is fatigued and that his or her abdomen is distended. Thanks to surgery and chemotherapy, the recovery rate among children suffering from nephroblastoma is more than 90 percent.

Nephrology: the science that focuses on the study of the kidneys and kidney-related diseases.

Nerve: the long whitish cords that in sections link our central nervous system to all the other parts of our body. Nerves are composed of fibrous tissues that function like electric wires, conveying sensitivity to the brain and excitation to the muscles (*see* "Central Nervous System," page 70).

Nerve fiber: a general term describing the microscopic structure of nerves.

Neuroblastoma: a cancer found most often in children aged less than ten years. Neuroblastoma can originate in the adrenal glands or the brain. Often, parents consult their doctor because the child is fatigued and excessively pale and, at times, suffers from violent headaches. Generally, neuroblastomas are life-threatening; often, at diagnosis, they have already produced metastases. The prognosis is better among children who have not yet reached the age of one. New treatment programs show very promising results.

Neurosurgery: a specialized form of surgery practiced on the central nervous system.

Neurology: the science that studies the brain and the nervous system.

Neutrophil: white cells belonging to the polynuclear family. Neutrophils play an important part in the body's fight against infection; if their number decreases (neutropenia), there is a major risk of infection.

Nucleus: the central part of the cell, containing all genetic information.

Obliterating bronchiolitis: an inflammation of the small bronchi, often linked to a graft versus host (GVH) reaction. The symptoms associated with bronchiolitis are coughing and shortness of breath. Its diagnosis often requires a biopsy of the lungs. Bronchiolitis is treated with cortisone.

Oncogene: a small portion of the genetic code that play a role in the development of a cancer.

Oncology: the science that focuses on the study of cancers and their treatment.

Opportunists: a term used to describe germs that infect an individual, particularly individuals suffering from immunodeficiency. The best-known germs of this type are microscopic fungi (candida albicans, aspergillus), microscopic parasites (pneumocystosis), and viruses.

Opportunistic infection: *see* Opportunist.

Osteolysis: the destruction of a portion of the bone as the result of an infectious, inflammatory, or cancerous phenomenon.

Osteopetrosis: a rare hereditary disease, characterized by an weakening and a thickening of the bones, resulting in repeated fractures and to blood-related problems. This disease is found in young children. A bone marrow transplant is the only treatment available for these patients (*see* "Congenital Diseases of the Blood," page 149).

Osteoporosis: a fragility of the bones, caused by a decrease in the quantity of calcium they contain. Osteoporosis occurs during cortisone-based treatment programs or after menopause.

Osteosarcoma: cancer of the bony tissue, frequently beginning with the long bones, such as the femur and the tibia. Osteosarcoma is most common among adolescents. The prognosis is poor. Treatment involves anticancer drugs and at times may also involve amputation of the affected limb.

Palliative treatment: a form treatment designed to decrease pain and to improve the patient's general condition, but without attacking the disease itself.

Paralysis: a nerve or central nervous system disorder that can make it impossible for one or more muscles to function properly.

Parasite: any living thing that depends on another to live; in hematology, doctors refer to microscopic parasites.

Parenteral feeding: method of administering food substitutes—such as proteins, sugars, and lipids—intravenously. Parenteral feeding is used when the patient is no longer able to eat food in the normal way.

Pelvis: large bone joining the spinal column to the lower limbs. The two upper parts of the pelvis are known as iliac; these areas are readily accessible and have bone marrow that is particularly rich in stem cells. Therefore, the pelvis is the ideal site for bone marrow samples (see "Bone Marrow," page 62).

Perfusion: the slow and prolonged introduction of liquids such as solutes, plasma, and certain drugs into the blood, intravenously.

Petechia: small red blotches caused by slight hemorrhages.

Phlebitis: the formation of a blood clot in a vein. Phlebitis is most common in lower limbs and is seen mainly in women, smokers, the obese, and bedridden or immobile individuals. The symptoms of phlebitis in a leg is swelling and sudden pain.

At times, the blood clot detaches and travels to the lungs; this condition is known as a pulmonary embolism and is considered to be a serious complication.

Philadelphia chromosome: an abnormal chromosome fond in the nuclei of leukemic cells in cases of chronic myelogenous leukemia.

Platelets: small cells that are found in the blood and whose main role is the formation of blood clots. The usual number of platelets is 150,000 to 400,000 per cubic millimeter.

Plasma: the liquid contained in the blood, composed of proteins, sugars, antibodies, and lipids.

Plasmapheresis: a technique using sophisticated equipment that separates plasma from blood cells. The equipment collects the plasma in a plastic bag and returns the blood cells to the patient's blood. Plasmapheresis is used for patients who receive a bone marrow transplant but who present an incompatibility with the donor's blood groups. It is also used to treat some diseases such as myeloma.

Plasmocytes: a type of white cells whose main characteristic is the ability to manufacture antibodies.

Pneumocystosis: an opportunistic parasite that infects the lungs of patients suffering from immunodeficiency. An antibiotic-based treatment program (Septra, Bactrim) prevents and cures this type of infection.

Pneumonia: a total or partial infection of the lung.

Potassium: a substance that is essential to the maintenance and work carried out by cells.

Prognosis: the doctor's forecast regarding a disease's progression and final result.

Prophylaxis: the measures taken to prevent infections (for example, proper hygiene, an extremely clean hospital room, antibiotics administered to prevent certain infections).

Proteins: a very complex class of molecules found in all human organs. There are hundreds of different proteins, all of which have a very specific job. In the blood, proteins such as hemoglobin, albumin, and antibodies are the best-known proteins.

Psychiatry: the branch of medicine that studies and treats stress-related problems and mental illness.

Psychosis: a mental problem involving the following problems: loss of contact with reality, strange behavior, incomprehensible conversation, irrational gestures. Psychoses can be caused by certain drugs or situations (for example, prolonged isolation) and are sometimes the result of mental illnesses such as schizophrenia.

Puberty: the passage from childhood to adolescence.

Pulmonary alveoli: small cavities found at the extremities of bronchi, whose function is to exchange air in the breathing process. While very small, the cavities are high in number; if all alveoli were removed from the lungs and spread out end to end, they would cover the equivalent of a football field (*see* Bronchi).

Pulmonary fibrosis: a thickening of the walls of pulmonary alveoli which hinders the circulation of oxygen and leads to progressive respiratory failure.

Puncture: a procedure used to collect liquid in a cavity or space.

Purging: a technique used in bone marrow transplants; it consists of removing the maximum number of cancer cells from the transplant recipient. The technique is practiced in a laboratory setting. The purified bone marrow can be reintroduced into the patient's system; this is known as an autologous transplant with selective depletion of cancerous cells.

Purpura: small hemorrhages characterized by the apparition of red blotches on the skin.

Rachicentesis: *see* Lumbar Puncture.

Radiation: the treatment of cancer through radiation.

Recurrence: a new manifestation of a disease that has been treated and that is considered as cured.

Regression: a patient's return to an earlier stage in the development of his or her disease. This term can also be used to describe a tumor that decreases in size.

Related donor: a person acting as a donor, who is directly related to the patient; for example, a brother or a sister.

Remission: the disappearance of all symptoms and all biological anomalies of a disease, following its treatment.

Renal failure: a decrease in the kidneys' functioning leading to a retention of liquids in the body and causing an accumulation of toxic wastes that can alter the work done by several other organs.

Retinoblastoma: cancer of the retina. Retinoblastoma is most common among children.

Retrovirus: a family of several types of viruses, including the AIDS virus.

Risk or risk factor: an epidemiological factor used to evaluate the probabilities that certain individuals will contract certain diseases. The risk is a useful factor in detecting subjects of groups. However, at least currently, the cause-and-effect link with the disease is not completely clear.

The risk factor is determined based on select observation groups. For example, groups of children can be compared to identify certain family-related and genetic risks, the presence of diseases that hinder the body's immune system and exposure to certain drugs and environmental factors that can increase the risk of contracting a form of leukemia.

Therefore, risk is a comparative value based on the value found in the general population; the closer an individual's risk is to the risk found in the general population, the more likely it is that the individual will remain healthy.

Glossary

Salivary glands: glands located close to the jaw, secreting saliva.

Sarcoma: a term used to describe cancers developed in certain types of tissues. Sarcomas are usually named after the tissues in which they have developed (osteosarcoma: cancer of the bones; lymphosarcoma: cancer of the lymph nodes).

Sciatica: pain originating in the lower back and irradiating to the buttocks and the calf of the leg. Sciatica is caused by an inflammation or a compression of the sciatic nerve.

Septicemia: a severe infections in which a germ infiltrates the blood. This type of infection must be treated promptly using high-dose antibiotics; otherwise, the patient may enter a state of shock.

Shingles: a skin infection causing painful irruptions. Shingles are caused by the Type 2 herpes virus, which also causes measles among children. The virus remains dormant in our nerves throughout our lifetime and causes shingles when reactivated. Shingles are most common among patients whose immune system is weakened and among elderly patients.

Shock: a sudden state of distress, characterized by a major drop in blood pressure. Patients turn pale, their hands and feet are cold, their breathing is quick; if the cause of shock are not eliminated quickly, neurological problems including coma can result. There are many causes leading to a state of shock; the most common are loss of blood due to hemorrhaging, severe infections with septicemia, heart failure, often linked to acute infarction, severe allergic reactions, or transfusional reactions. In all instances, to prevent neurological problems, the state of shock must be alleviated quickly.

Solute: a liquid containing sugars and minerals, administered to patients intravenously. Solutes are packaged in plastic bags containing 250, 500, or 1,000 cubic centimeters.

Spermatogenesis: the formation of sperm in the testicles.

Spleen: an organ located on the left side of the abdomen. The spleen stocks and destroys old red cells. It also generates certain types of white cells. A few diseases—such as mononucleosis, leukemia, and lymphomas—can cause the spleen to increase in size and can make it vulnerable to the slightest impact.

Splenectomy: a surgical procedure to remove the spleen.

Splenomegaly: the condition of a spleen that has increased in size. There are many causes underlying splenomegaly: the most common are viral (mononucleosis) and bacterial (endocarditis) infections, cancers (leukemia, lymphoma), and severe liver disease.

Spontaneous remission: a remission that occurs without treatment. Spontaneous remission is a disappearance of the signs of a disease, with scientifically based explanation. In the case of malignant blood diseases, spontaneous remissions are extremely rare.

Stem cells: cells that are found in the bone marrow; they have the ability to multiply and they generate all of the cells found in the blood. These are precious cells and are life-giving in instances of bone marrow transplants.

Sterility: a living being's inability to reproduce.

Sternum: a flat bone located in the center of the thorax. The sternum contains bone marrow that is rich is stem cells.

Survival rate: the ratio expressing the number of patients who recover following treatment. The recovery rate is expressed as a percentage.

Symptom: a manifestation of a disease that can be perceived by patients themselves (for example: coughing, fever, and greenish spittle are symptoms of pneumonia).

Syndrome: the symptoms and clinical signs a patient presents, but not a true disease.

Often, a new disease is described as a syndrome because its causes and manifestations are not well known. Thanks to research, doctors can arrive at a better understanding of a given syndrome and, at this point, it is described as a disease. The acquired immunodeficiency syndrome (AIDS) is a well-known example.

Tear glands: glands that secrete tears.

Thalassemia: a form of anemia that is transmitted genetically and that exists in two forms: a major form, that is very serious, and a minor form, in which subjects present few symptoms.

Thrombosis: an obliteration of a blood vessel, arterial or venous. The most common cause of thrombosis is arteriosclerosis (fatty deposits in arteries).

Glossary

Tissue: a word used to describe a group of cells that have the same function; for example, a nerve is composed of nerve tissue.

Transfusional reaction: a series of symptoms (fever, shivering, trembling) present in a patient who receives a transfusion of blood products (red cells, platelets, plasma). Transfusional reactions are caused by the presence of antibodies in the blood of a patient who receives a transfusion. These antibodies are directed against the transfused products. As soon as symptoms appear, the transfusion is stopped.

Transfusional reactions must always be monitored closely.

Treatment program: the measures taken to treat a patient, designed to achieve the patient's recovery while maintaining the best possible quality of life.

Trisomy or Down's syndrome: a congenital disease characterized by learning difficulties, a round and wide face, and slanted eyes. Children with Down's syndrome often present malformations of the heart and digestive system. Down's syndrome is caused by an abnormality in chromosome 21. The risk of having a child with Down's syndrome is higher when women give birth after the age of thirty-five.

Tumor: a clump of cells forming a lump. Doctors recognize two types of tumors: benign tumors, which are delimited and do not invade adjacent organs, and malignant tumors, or cancers, which tend to invade adjacent organs.

Ultrasonography: a technique used to explore the organs, based on ultrasound reflection. The ultrasonograph is painless and does not jeopardize the patient's health in any way.

Unit of blood: a quantity of blood equivalent to approximately 500 cubic centimeters or a pint.

Unrelated donor: a person acting as a donor who is not related to the patient in any way.

Uric acid: an acid usually produced in small quantities by the liver, kidneys, and intestines. The destruction of cancerous cells can result in an increase in the amount of uric acid found in the blood, and the acid can form tiny crystals. The accumulation of uric acid crystals can damage the kidneys and can cause joint pain.

Urine output: the amount of urine produced by the kidneys. Over a twenty-four-hour period, for individuals in good health, the average is one quart to one quart and a half.

Veins: blood vessels that carry blood from all parts of the body to the heart. Blood found in veins is blue in color.

Vertebral canal: a space located in the back, running along the center of the spinal column. The vertebral canal contains the spinal cord, which is surrounded by a liquid known as cerebrospinal fluid.

Virus: very small germs that cannot be seen through a standard microscope; viruses can be seen only through electronic microscopes that can magnify several thousands of times. Viruses are detected by looking for their antibodies in the patient's blood. There are hundreds of different viruses, the most common of which are the following:

Table of Viruses and Associated Diseases

Virus	*Associated disease*
Influenza	Severe cold
Epstein-Barr	Mononucleosis
Herpes Simplex II	Shingles
Human immunodeficiency virus	AIDS
Cytomegalovirus	Severe pneumonia

White mouth: an infection of the mouth characterized by white blotches caused by a microscopic fungus known as candida albicans.

References and Suggested Reading

Altman, R. and M. J. Sarg. *The Cancer Dictionary*. New York: Facts on File, 1992.

Armitage, J.O. *Bone Marrow Transplantation*. Omaha: Medical Progress, vol. 330, no. 12.

Bennet, J.C. et al (eds.). *Cecil Textbook of Medicine*. Philadelphia: Saunders, 1996.

Cancer Medicine. Department of Continuing Education, divison of Medical Oncology, Dana Farber Cancer Institute, Harvard Medical School, 1989.

De Vita, V.T., S. Hellman, and S. Rosenburg. *Cancer: Principles and Practice of Oncology*. Philadelphia: Lippincott-Raven, 1997.

Dollinger, M. and E.H. Rosenbaum. *Everyone's Guide to Cancer Therapy: How Cancer Is Diagnosed, Treated and Managed Day to Day*, 3rd ed. Kansas City, MO: Andrews and McMeel, 1997.

Holland, J.F. et al (eds.) *Cancer Medicine*, 4th ed. Baltimore: Williams and Wilkins, 1997.

Isselbacher, K.J. et al. *Principals of Internal Medicine*. New York: McGraw-Hill, 1994.

McAllister, R.M. *Cancer*. New York: Basic Books, 1993.

Millev, D. *Blood Diseases of Infancy and Childhood*, 6th ed. Mosby, 1989.

Pazdur, P. *Medical Oncology: A Comprehensive Review*. Huntington, NY: PRR, 1995